Practical
Genetic Counselling

by Peter S Harper MA DM FRCP

Reader and Consultant in Medical Genetics,
Welsh National School of Medicine and
University Hospital of Wales, Cardiff

Bristol
John Wright & Sons Ltd
1981

© **P. S. Harper,**
   University Hospital of Wales, Heath Park, Cardiff, CF4 4XW. 1981.

Published by
John Wright & Sons Ltd, 42–44 Triangle West, Bristol, BS8 1EX.

First published, 1981
Reprinted, 1982

British Library Cataloguing in Publication Data

   Harper, Peter S
      Practical genetic counselling.
      1. Medical genetics
      I. Title
      616′.042   RB155

ISBN 0 7236 0567 X

Printed in Great Britain by
John Wright & Sons (Printing) Ltd, at The Stonebridge Press, Bristol, BS4 5NU

To
Elaine
and to
Matthew
Emma Jane
Nicholas
and
Katy Thi

Preface

During the period of almost 10 years in which I have been running a medical genetics clinic and service, many people have asked me to recommend a simple book to help them in giving genetic counselling. Most of these have been fellow clinicians, chiefly paediatricians and more recently, obstetricians, faced in their regular practice with inherited or possibly inherited disorders and wishing to provide patients and their families with accurate information. Increasing public awareness and the possibility in some instances of prenatal diagnosis has increased the importance of such information being readily available.

Until now, I have been unable to recommend fully any book of this type, though numerous detailed works exist on specific groups of inherited disorders, as well as excellent introductory books on human genetics. Indeed, it may be asked whether a single book can any longer cover the amount of detailed information that is relevant to genetic counselling without danger of being superficial and inaccurate. Such dangers are real, but nevertheless, I believe firmly that such a book is needed and after waiting in vain for my colleagues to provide it, have attempted to do so myself.

I should emphasize from the outset that this book is written primarily for practising clinicians, whether in family practice or hospital specialties. It does not attempt to provide the extent or depth of information needed for the medical geneticist running a genetic counselling clinic; however I suspect that even my more erudite colleagues would find a simple book useful for those not infrequent occasions when one's memory lapses and there is no immediate access to more detailed literature. I can think of many occasions when I would have appreciated such a book. A further group who may find it useful is the increasing number of paramedical and non-medical staff associated with medical genetics centres and their allied laboratory services.

In writing this book, I owe a considerable debt to many people. Perhaps the greatest is to my former teachers, Professor E. B. Ford, Sir Cyril Clarke and Dr Victor McKusick of Oxford, Liverpool and Baltimore respectively, who not only fired my enthusiasm for the subject, but who influenced my conception of what medical genetics should be, and in particular how it could remain closely linked to clinical practice without losing its scientific basis.

More immediately, I must thank all my colleagues in Cardiff for their suggestions, criticism and support. Special thanks are also due to Professor Cedric Carter, Professor Alan Emery, Dr Rodney Harris and Dr Ian Young for their detailed comments on the entire manuscript, which resulted in a number of errors being corrected and in other sections being extensively rewritten. I should be glad to be notified of any remaining errors or omissions, or indeed of any suggestions for improvement, since I hope to keep the book updated at regular intervals.

Finally, I should like to thank the Department of Medical Illustration of the Welsh National School of Medicine for redrawing most of the pedigrees, Mrs Edna Long and Mrs Julie Kruydenburg for typing and checking the manuscript, and John Wright & Sons Ltd of Bristol and W. B. Saunders of Philadelphia for their helpful and efficient role in its publication.

Cardiff, 1980   P.S.H.

Contents

I. General Aspects of Genetic Counselling

CHAPTER ONE

Genetic Counselling: an Introduction

Although most people working in the field of medicine are familiar with the term 'genetic counselling', and have some idea as to what it means, it is surprisingly rare to see the term actually defined. Closer enquiry among patients and colleagues shows a wide variation in people's concepts of what the process of genetic counselling actually entails. Some envisage an essentially supportive, even psychotherapeutic role, akin to that of counselling processes in the social field; others see genetic counselling as primarily concerned with special diagnostic tests in inherited disease; others again regard it as a complex mathematical process in working out risk estimates.

All these views of genetic counselling contain an element of truth, but all are wide of the mark in identifying what the process of genetic counselling actually involves. Even within the group of professionals for whom genetic counselling is a major activity there are varied opinions as to its proper role and scope, but the following definition includes what the author believes to be the essential features.

'Genetic counselling is the process by which patients or relatives at risk of a disorder that may be hereditary are advised of the consequences of the disorder, the probability of developing and transmitting it and of the ways in which this may be prevented or ameliorated'.

From this definition it can be seen that all three aspects mentioned in the opening paragraph are indeed involved – a diagnostic aspect, without which all advice has an insecure foundation; the actual estimation of risks, which may be simple in some situations and complex in others; and a supportive role ensuring that those given advice actually benefit from it and from the various preventive measures that may be available. This chapter outlines the main steps in this process, which are then dealt with in more detail in subsequent sections of the book. It is the satisfactory synthesis of these various aspects which makes up genetic counselling as a specific process.

The Development of Genetic Counselling

The study of human genetics was already well developed by the early decades of the present century; Charles Davenport of the Eugenics Records Office in New York State began to give genetic advice as early as 1910.

However, genetic counselling did not emerge as a recognized procedure until much later. During the 1920s and 1930s the development of 'eugenic' policies in both totalitarian Germany and in N. America, accompanied by discriminatory laws prohibiting marriage of those with particular diseases, brought the subject of eugenics into disrepute; it was not until the time of the Second World War that the first genetic counselling clinics were opened in America, in Michigan (1940) and Minnesota (1941)[1]. In the UK the Hospital for Sick Children in Great Ormond Street, London, developed the first such clinic in 1946. By 1955 there were over a dozen centres in N. America and a steady development has occurred since that time; the current National Foundation directory[2] lists 450 centres in N. America and 40 in the UK. As with many pioneering developments, the early centres were often the work of far-sighted eccentrics. Sheldon Reed, in his book *Counselling in Medical Genetics,* first published in 1955[3], gives a delightful description of Edward Dight, responsible for founding the Dight Clinic in Minneapolis, who lived in a house built in a tree and who failed to file income tax returns. Francis Galton, who originated what was to become the Galton Laboratory in London, was another, though more scientific individualist.

Reed's book gives a vivid picture of the main areas covered in the early stages of genetic counselling, and it was Reed himself who first introduced the term. Many of the problems are unchanged today and his examples of individual cases show that the fears and concerns of families have altered little. In other respects there have been profound changes in the 25 years since the book was written. Carrier detection was almost non-existent and prenatal diagnosis entirely so, so the options open to patients at risk were limited; either they took the risk or they did not. An even more important change has been that of the general climate of opinion among the public and the medical profession.

Reed's case histories illustrate the background of ignorance and prejudice which his patients had to cope with and it is no wonder that he found them grateful, even when he could only give them pessimistic advice.

It is of interest that the commonest cause of referral to the Dight clinic was regarding skin colour and whether a child for adoption would 'pass for white'. Several other problems among the 20 commonest causes for referral listed by Reed are infrequently encountered today, including eye colour, twinning and rhesus haemolytic disease. The last of these provides a real example of advance in treatment and prevention; the others reflect changes in social attitudes. Many others of Reed's commonest problems remain equally important today, including mental subnormality, schizophrenia, facial clefting, neural tube defects and Huntington's chorea.

Constructing a Family Tree

Collecting genetic information is the first and most important step in genetic counselling, and is best achieved by drawing up a family tree or pedigree. The use of clear and consistent symbols allows genetic information to be set out much more clearly than does a long list of relatives. Drawing a satisfactory pedigree is not difficult, though it is remarkable how rarely those clinicians without an interest in genetics will attempt the process! A clearly drawn pedigree has a certain aesthetic appeal, but its chief value is to provide an unambiguous and permanent record of the genetic information in a particular family.

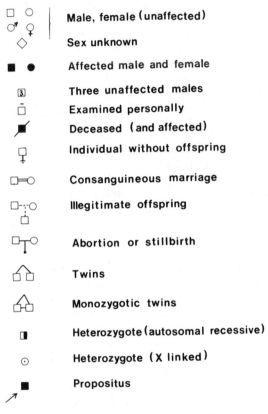

Fig. 1.1. Symbols used in drawing a pedigree.

Fig. 1.1 shows the main symbols used in constructing pedigrees, some of which are briefly explained. The symbols shown for the sexes (□, ○) are preferred to the alternative ♂ and ♀ symbols, which tend to be confused at a distance. Heterozygous carriers can be denoted by half-shaded symbols, or in the case of an X-linked disorder by a central dot. Although the sign for an early abortion can also be used for a stillbirth it is preferable to denote the sex with an appropriate symbol and indicate that it was a stillbirth beneath.

The *proband* or *propositus* (female *proposita*) should be clearly indicated with an arrow. The proband is the individual (or individuals) through whom the family is ascertained. Large families will commonly have several probands. The proband is generally an affected individual, but the person primarily seeking advice may well not be affected. The term '*consultand*' is conveniently used for this individual.

Multiple marriages and complex consanguinity can cause problems in constructing a pedigree, and artistry will have to be sacrificed for accuracy in such cases. It is usually wise to start near the middle of one's pedigree sheet and to leave more room than one thinks will be needed, so that particularly prolific family branches do not become crowded out. *Fig.* 1.2 shows examples of a simple and more complex 'working pedigree'. The following practical points deserve emphasis.

1. Enquire specifically about the infant deaths, stillbirths and abortions. These may be highly relevant and the fact that they have not been volunteered may be significant. Thus two children 'lost at birth' by the mother of a woman seen for counselling proved both to have had spina bifida, a fact which considerably altered the risks.

2. Consanguinity should be directly asked about and may be the clue which suggests autosomal recessive inheritance.

3. Illegitimacy must be borne in mind, especially in a puzzling situation. A family doctor or nurse may well, particularly in a small community, be able to clarify this possibility. Illegitimacy is not of course the problem, but mistaken paternity.

4. Always take at least basic details about both sides of the family, even in a dominantly inherited disorder clearly originating from one side. Unexpected findings may emerge. The family that insists that there is 'nothing on our side' should be regarded with suspicion until this is verified. Taking details about both sides may also help to avoid feelings of guilt or blame resting exclusively on one member of a couple.

5. Record dates of birth where possible rather than ages. Note the date when the pedigree was drawn up.

6. Record maiden names of women; this is especially significant for X-linked disorders, where the surname of affected members is likely to change with each generation.

7. Note the addresses of relevant members — this may prove invaluable in obtaining hospital records or in later contact with relatives.

Most of the above points are obvious, yet it is surprising how often initial information is not obtained unless a systematic approach is used.

Diagnostic Information

It has already been emphasized that a clear diagnosis is the essential basis for accurate genetic counselling. Unfortunately, this basis is all too often a

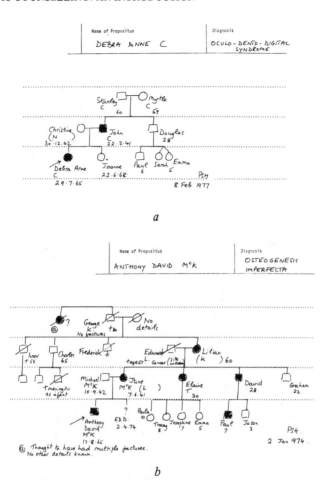

Fig. 1.2. Two examples of the 'working pedigree'. These two pedigrees, one simple, the other more extensive, show how family data can be easily but clearly recorded at the time of interview. A simple lined sheet is used; more detailed information on individuals can be recorded at the foot of the pedigree sheet or on the back.

shaky one, and one of the principal tasks of anyone involved in genetic counselling is to ensure that it is made as firm as possible before risk estimates are given to those seeking advice. Common reasons for lack of a clear diagnosis include the following:

1. *The affected individual may have lived a considerable time ago, when relevant diagnostic investigations were not available.* There is little that can be done about this, but it is surprising how much detailed information may be obtained by questioning close relatives who were involved

in caring for the patient. Even if an exact diagnosis cannot be established, it may be possible to *exclude* a disorder. Thus a man with 'muscular dystrophy' who lived to the age of 40 clearly did not have the Duchenne type.

2. *The affected individual may have died without essential investigations having been done, or without autopsy being performed.* This is all too often the case and is inexcusable. Reasons usually offered are reluctance to trouble the parents in distressing circumstances, or the fact that investigations will not alter the patient's management, but usually the real reason is that those involved have not taken the trouble to undertake the studies, nor to make arrangements with those who can undertake them. The tragic consequences of such inertia only become apparent when the question of risk to further family members arises.

3. *A firm diagnosis cannot be reached even with the affected individual living.* This is inevitable in some cases, since our knowledge of many genetic disorders remains very incomplete, but a considerable degree of help can be obtained by enlisting the efforts of colleagues, even at a distance. Photographs, X-rays, urine, blood and cultured skin fibroblast samples can all be sent to distant parts of the world for experts to study, and presentation of puzzling cases at clinical meetings may often result in a diagnosis being provided. Even if it does not, one can feel happier that one is not overlooking a recognizable disorder if one has sought the advice of those most likely to know.

4. *The diagnosis may be wrong.* This is a much more dangerous situation than when the diagnosis is uncertain, for it may lead to false confidence. It is extremely difficult to know how far to rely on other people's diagnoses and how far to insist on confirming them oneself. Clearly neither a medical geneticist, nor any other clinician, can be an expert diagnostician in every specialty, and one will frequently have to rely on colleagues' advice; nevertheless it is essential for anyone involved in genetic counselling to have a wide range of diagnostic ability, to know his limitations – and those of his colleagues – and to develop a healthy scepticism in diagnostic matters and a sensitivity for where error may lie.

Bearing in mind the foregoing problems, how can the clinician involved in genetic counselling ensure that his diagnostic information is as extensive and accurate as may be? There is no simple answer, but the following points may be helpful.

1. Always arrange to see the affected individual or individuals where possible, even if they have already been fully investigated. How detailed an examination is required will depend on circumstances.

2. Always examine asymptomatic members at risk to exclude mild or early disease. This is especially important with variable dominantly inherited disorders or where there is a possibility of new mutation.

3. Warn families in advance that the full answers to their questions may not be possible on the initial visit, and ask them to bring as much

relevant information as possible about affected individuals, especially those not in the same household as themselves.

4. Be prepared to interview older or more distant relatives who may have valuable information on deceased individuals. A home visit may be very useful here. Such relatives will almost always be happy to help, but the part of the family requesting advice should be told beforehand that other branches are going to be approached and asked whether any members are likely to be upset by this.

5. When arranging a follow-up appointment for counselling, allow adequate time for obtaining records and other information.

6. A variety of special investigations may prove necessary, including radiology, biochemical and cytogenetic studies and sometimes biopsy diagnosis. Most studies can be done on an outpatient basis, but it is extremely helpful to have facilities for inpatient investigation. It frequently happens that the affected individual on whom investigations are needed is already under the care of a clinical colleague; obviously careful liaison prior to seeing such a person is essential if confusion or duplication of investigations is to be avoided and good working relationships with colleagues maintained.

Risks and Odds

Having taken a careful pedigree, documented the various details of affected individuals and examined relevant family members, one is now in a position to actually attempt to answer the questions which gave rise to the request for genetic counselling and to estimate and transmit to the family concerned the risks of particular members, born or unborn, developing the particular disorder. The fact that the process of recording information will probably have taken a considerable time is in some ways an advantage, particularly if the family is not under one's regular care but is being seen specifically for counselling. From the way in which information is given (or not given) and from the reaction to questions, a lot can be learned about the general attitude of the individuals being counselled to the family disorder: Did they themselves initiate the request for counselling or not? Is there an unspoken and perhaps exaggerated fear of the disorder? Do feelings of guilt or hostility between parents exist? Is the rest of the family supportive or has it aggravated the situation? Is an affected child valued and loved or regarded as an intolerable burden?

It is also possible during this preliminary stage to assess the way in which information is to be most suitably transmitted. Some couples will be unable to grasp more than the simplest concepts of 'high' or 'low risk', while others will require a precise risk figure and even a detailed explanation of the mode of inheritance.

Information on genetic risks is rarely an absolute 'yes' or 'no', and in medical genetics, more perhaps than in any other branch of medicine, one thinks and works almost entirely in terms of *probabilities* or *odds*.

Colleagues frequently find this unsatisfactory, preferring to accept only a 'definite' conclusion. Yet when examined closely there is often as much if not more uncertainty in the apparently 'definite' specialties as there is in medical genetics. Thus the chance that a definitely inflamed appendix will be found at appendicectomy is far from 100 per cent, while the entire process of clinical diagnosis is based on the combination of numerous

Table 1.1. Risk estimates. Conversion table between odds and percentages

Odds	%	%	Odds
1 in 2	50	50	1 in 2
3	33	40	2·5
4	25	30	3·3
5	20	25	4
6	17	20	5
7	14	15	6·7
8	12	12	8·3
9	11	10	10
10	10	9	11
12	8	8	12·5
14	7	7	14
16	6	6	17
18	5·5	5	20
20	5·0	4	25
25	4·0	3	33
30	3·3	3	50
35	2·9	1	100
40	2·5	0·5	200
50	2·0	0·25	400
60	1·7	0·1	1000
70	1·4		
80	1·3		
90	1·1		
100	1·0		

pieces of information, each with a degree of uncertainty, though this is often unappreciated by those involved. The same applies to the 'normal ranges' of most laboratory investigations. It is perhaps only because uncertainty is well recognized in genetics that methods of measuring it and defining its limits have become generally used, as exemplified in genetic counselling.

Risk figures in genetic counselling may be given either as odds or as percentages. Some people prefer to use odds and to quote risks as 1 in 10, 1 in 50, 1 in 100, etc. Others prefer to use such figures as 10 per cent, 2 per cent, 1 per cent. The author admits to inconsistency in this, both in practice and in this book, and for this reason, and because others are equally inconsistent, a table of conversions is given (*Table* 1.1) which should allow ready exchange between the two approaches. It is often necessary to adapt which one uses to a particular counselling situation, for some people simply do not understand odds, while others are more confused with percentages.

Whatever method one uses, there are pitfalls in interpretation which must be avoided, and this may require much patience.

1. Odds refer to the future, not the past. Thus in a situation of 1 in 4 risk, as seen with autosomal recessive inheritance, this does *not* mean that the fact that the previous child was affected guarantees the next three being normal. Nor does having two affected children in succession make it less (or more) likely that the next will be affected. That 'chance has no memory' may require repeated explanation.

2. It is embarrassingly easy for odds to be reversed. Thus a patient seen by the author with one spina bifida child, having been correctly advised by her obstetrician that there was a 1 in 20 recurrence risk, came seeking termination in her next pregnancy because she considered that 'a chance of 1 in 20 of a normal child was far too low!'

3. Odds of 1 *in* 2 are not the same as 1 *to* 2; this may be misinterpreted by those used to betting. Fortunately, the difference is only considerable for the highest risks.

4. Many people do not have a clear idea of what constitutes a 'high' or 'low risk'. Thus some couples who are given a low risk (e.g. 1 in 200) express the view that this is far too high to be acceptable, whereas others seen by the author have been greatly relieved by a risk of 50 per cent. Clearly the nature of the disorder will determine what risk is acceptable, but it is helpful to be able to give some kind of reference point for comparison, such as the fact that 1 child in 30 in the population is born with a significant handicap, or that the population frequency of the disorder in question is (say) 1 in 2000. Some useful data of this type are summarized in *Table* 1.2.

Table 1.2. Risk of abnormalities in the 'normal' population

Risk of a child being born with some congenital abnormality	1 in 30
Risk of a child being born with a serious physical or mental handicap	1 in 50
Risk of a pregnancy ending in a spontaneous abortion	1 in 8
Risk of perinatal death*	1 in 30 to 1 in 100
Risk of a child dying in the first year of life after first week*	1 in 150
Risk that a couple will be infertile	1 in 10

*Figures for 'developed' countries; great variation between regions.

The Estimation of Risks
The ways in which risks can be estimated and the results of these estimates form the basis of this book and are considered in detail in later chapters.

It is important from the outset, though, to recognize that not all risk estimates are of the same type. They may be based on different sorts of information and may be of greater or lesser reliability. The following main categories can be recognized:

1. *Empiric risks* (*Fig.* 1.3) (*see* Chapter 3). Here the estimate is based on observed data rather than theoretical predictions; this is the form of risk estimate available for most of the commoner non-Mendelian or chromosomal disorders. The information is usually reliable provided it has been collected in an unbiased manner (often not easy) and provided that the population from which the individual receiving counselling comes is comparable to the one on which the data were established.

Fig. 1.3. Empiric risk estimate. One child is affected with spina bifida. The risk of a subsequent child being affected by a neural tube defect is 1 in 20 in a high risk area (e.g. South Wales) and with no other affected family members. The risk estimate would be different in a low incidence area and would be altered by the presence of other affected relatives.

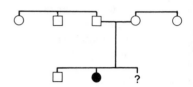

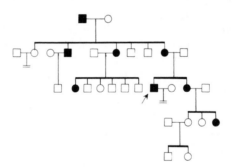

Fig. 1.4. Mendelian risk estimate. A family with myotonic dystrophy (an autosomal dominant disorder). The risk for the offspring of affected individuals is 50 per cent regardless of the incidence of the disorder and the number of affected individuals in the family.

2. *Mendelian risks* (*Fig.* 1.4) (*see* Chapter 2). These can only be given when a clear basis of Mendelian inheritance can be recognized for a disorder. They are perhaps the most satisfactory form of risk estimate since they commonly allow a clear differentation into categories of negligible risk (e.g. offspring of healthy sibs in an autosomal recessive disorder) and

high risk (e.g. offspring of an individual affected with an autosomal dominant disorder). There often remains the problem of achieving greater certainty in the individual at high risk (e.g. a person at 50 per cent risk of developing Huntington's chorea), and information from the next two categories may be helpful in this situation.

3. *Modified genetic risks (Fig. 1.5).* Non-geneticists may find this type of estimate difficult to use initially; it is particularly applicable in X-linked recessive inheritance, where fully worked out examples are given (*see* Chapters 2 and 5). The essential feature is that a 'prior' genetic risk, based

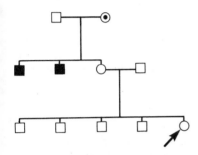

Fig. 1.5. Modified risk estimate. Duchenne muscular dystrophy. The grandmother of the individual seeking advice (consultand) is an obligatory carrier; and prior risks of the mother and the consultand being carriers are thus 50 per cent and 25 per cent respectively. These risks are, however, greatly reduced by the fact that the mother has had four healthy and no affected sons (*see* Chapter 2 for further details).

usually on Mendelian inheritance, may be modified by 'conditional' information, usually genetic, but sometimes from other sources. Thus the modified risk of a man developing Huntington's chorea whose grandparent was affected is not the same as the prior risk of 1 in 4, but is reduced by his own age and by that of the intervening unaffected parent. It may also be reduced by the number of unaffected sibs, if these have reached an advanced age. Such modifying information may drastically alter the risk estimate and should always be used when available.

4. *Risk estimates from independent evidence.* Where special investigations can be utilized these may greatly alter the risk estimates. Thus a normal amniotic fluid alphafetoprotein in a pregnancy of a woman who has one child with a neural tube defect will reduce the risk of an affected child from 1 in 20 to around 1 in 200. Carrier detection in such disorders as haemophilia and Duchenne muscular dystrophy provides comparable information. However, a strong caution must be given here: the results of these investigations are rarely so clear cut that they can be used in isolation; they require combination with the prior genetic risk, along with other modifying information. Failure to appreciate this may lead to serious error, especially when investigations are being applied as screening procedures in situations of low prior risk. Examples of this are given in Chapter 5.

5. *Composite risks.* Most empiric risks really fall into this category, but in some instances it is obvious that one is dealing with a mixed situation

which cannot be satisfactorily resolved. Thus a disorder such as osteogenesis imperfecta congenita may be composed of a large number of cases representing new dominant mutations, with negligible recurrence risk to sibs, and a small number of autosomal recessive cases, with a recurrence risk of 1 in 4. Since the two forms cannot at present be reliably distinguished, one ends up with an intermediate risk depending on the relative frequency of the two groups. Obviously this intermediate risk does not really exist at all – the family must represent one or other of the extreme positions. Such a composite risk estimate is an unsatisfactory one and should be regarded as a temporary measure. With improved resolution of genetic heterogeneity it may be possible to distinguish the individual components, while even within a single family additional information may resolve the situation. Thus the birth of a further affected child in the example given of osteogenesis imperfecta would make it almost certain that autosomal recessive inheritance is operating in this family, with a 1 in 4 risk for further children.

'Directive' Genetic Counselling

It will have been noted that the emphasis so far has been placed on ensuring that a correct diagnosis and risk estimate have been reached and that those being counselled have correctly understood the situation. Nothing has been said about advising a particular line of action or of recommending couples against having children in high risk situations, and it may surprise readers to learn that the author, in common with most clinicians involved in genetic counselling, rarely adopts a 'directive' approach.

This situation may appear all the more surprising since many doctors with little experience of genetics do frequently give directive advice. Remarks such as 'we were told not to have further children' or 'the doctors said I must have it terminated' are commonly heard at a genetic counselling clinic, and in many cases great distress has been caused to the couples involved, especially since the advice has rarely been accompanied by an explanation of why it has been given or how great the risk really is.

The author's view is that it is not the duty of a doctor to order the lives of others, but to ensure that individuals have the facts to enable them to make their own decisions. This includes not simply a knowledge of the genetic risks, but a clear appreciation of the consequences, long as well as short term, which may result from a particular course of action. In any case, it seems likely, though not proven, that directive counselling may be counterproductive. Intelligent couples may resent being told what to do in a situation where they have already spent much troubled thought over the alternatives. Among the less privileged there is often a strong resentment of being dictated to by authority and the author's experience with Huntington's chorea suggests that some individuals in this situation may deliberately embark on a pregnancy as a gesture of defiance.

By contrast, some couples seen for genetic counselling will plead for direction. 'What would you do if you were in my place?' is a common question. It is tempting to give a clear direction in these circumstances, but frequently these are the very couples where this may be most inadvisable. Such a plea often indicates an unwillingness to face up to the consequences of a serious situation, or a serious disagreement between marriage partners, and for the physician to take on the responsibility that can only really be taken by the couple themselves may have serious long-term consequences.

It would be wrong to pretend that those engaged in genetic counselling never give directive advice. One's own views are likely to be expressed in the way one approaches the subject, whether one has stressed the more serious or the milder aspects of a disease and whether one holds out the possibility of future treatment. Even the way one phrases a risk estimate can vary — thus in an autosomal recessive situation with a 1 in 4 recurrence risk it is possible to make it appear quite encouraging if one states that there are three chances out of four that the child will be healthy!

The only disorder where the author is consciously directive in his advice is Huntington's chorea. Here the long-term consequences of the disease are so disastrous for a family that it seems reasonable to encourage those at 50 per cent risk to avoid childbearing or at least to limit their family. Even here, though, if couples make a clear decision to go ahead with reproduction, one must respect their wishes.

Genetic Counselling 'by Proxy'

The less one is able to verify a situation personally, the greater is the possibility of error. However, the person who refuses to give any advice unless able to do everything himself is going to be of limited benefit to his patients and his colleagues. The author is in no doubt that one of the most valuable roles of a medical geneticist — and the same applies to any clinician with a particular interest in genetic counselling — is to act as a focal point and source of information for colleagues in a variety of specialties who need someone to turn to for advice. A high proportion of telephone and postal enquiries from colleagues do not require actual referral of the patient; frequently one is simply confirming what is already thought to be the case, in other instances one may be able to advise that prenatal or other special investigations are available; in a small proportion, however, the advice has to be that one cannot give a reliable opinion without seeing the full situation for oneself.

Actual genetic counselling by post or other indirect means is an entirely different matter, and the author's policy regarding enquiries from patients and relatives is to arrange a clinic appointment, via their family doctor wherever possible. The same policy applies to enquiries from health visitors, social workers and other paramedical personnel. Not only is there

a serious risk that erroneous information may be given or risk figures misinterpreted, but without directly seeing those requesting advice it is often
impossible to decide what the real problem leading to their enquiry is and
whether there are additional or underlying factors that have not been
mentioned.

The Back-up to Genetic Counselling

It has already been emphasized that genetic counselling does not simply
consist of giving risk figures, and that it must often be preceded by a
considerable diagnostic effort, in comparison with which the estimation
of risks may be a relatively simple matter. Similarly, genetic counselling
does not stop with the giving of risks but must include a variety of other
actions if it is to be fully effective.

In the first instance, it must be established as clearly as possible that the
individuals counselled have really understood what has been told them.
This includes not only the risk estimate, but the nature of the disorder
and what other measures are available for prevention and treatment. It is
often possible to get an approximate idea of how well information has
been understood at the time of the interview, but it is well worthwhile,
and often a salutary experience, to have this checked by an independent
observer. A skilled social worker can often do this while discussing other
matters with the family after the consultation, and will surprisingly often
find that part or all of the information has been forgotten or misinterpreted before the couple has even left the clinic. A system of regular
follow-up is useful both to check on this and to reinforce the counselling
that has been given at the initial interview. For the same reason, it may be
helpful to give couples a summary or diagram to illustrate the risks,
though this has not been the author's regular practice.

Where information has been seriously misinterpreted or forgotten this
may be for various reasons. Some individuals have genuinely poor memories,
others may have been seen at an inappropriate time, such as soon after the
death of a child. Yet others have come to the clinic encumbered with small
and active children and have been preoccupied in restraining their activities
rather than in listening to what one has said. Most commonly, one has
probably not taken sufficient time and effort to ensure that the information has really been absorbed and it is important to be aware of one's
failures in this respect. The author has on several occasions seen couples
who have acquired grossly erroneous ideas of risks and has wondered who
could possibly have misinformed them so completely, only to find that
he has seen them himself some years previously!

An essential accompaniment to genetic counselling is that those being
counselled should have full and accurate knowledge of the various preventive measures that may be available. In many cases these require
application as an integral part of counselling — thus an assessment of the

risk of a woman having a child affected by Duchenne muscular dystrophy or haemophilia is incomplete without undertaking tests of carrier detection (Chapter 5). In other cases the risk may not be altered, but the consequences may be. Thus, where prenatal diagnosis is available (Chapter 6), many couples will be prepared to embark on a high-risk pregnancy when they would not have considered doing so in the absence of this. Similarly, the development of treatment fundamentally alters attitudes to genetic counselling. Many couples with a phenylketonuric child diagnosed in the newborn period and developing normally with treatment are happy to risk another affected child; where treatment is less satisfactory and the outcome less certain the attitude may be very different.

Further 'back-up' measures that may be required are contraception and sterilization as well as the exploration of other possible options such as adoption and artificial insemination by donor. These aspects are discussed later (Chapter 8) but it cannot be too strongly emphasized that their consideration is an integral part of genetic counselling.

Finally, many couples coming for genetic counselling require active support in one way or another. Sometimes the actual information given in genetic counselling may be of such serious consequence as to require support if serious problems are not to arise. Huntington's chorea (Chapter 10) is perhaps the most striking example, but a severe depressive reaction is not uncommon in women who have recently lost a child after a chronic illness and have to be told that the risk for other children is high. A sympathetic family doctor to whom the couple can turn is probably the best safeguard in this situation, but a skilled social worker can often accurately judge those families especially needing support.

Support may also be required for problems quite unrelated to the genetic aspects. Thus in genetic counselling for a chronic disease, it is frequently found that an affected individual is receiving no medical attention at all, that practical aids such as wheelchairs are not being provided, or that social service benefits of various kinds are not being claimed. It is sometimes argued that such matters are not part of genetic counselling; this may theoretically be so, but as a physician the author feels strongly that genetic counselling is an integral part of the overall management of a patient and his family, that basic supportive measures may be as important or even more so than the actual information regarding genetic risks, and that it is one's duty to see the necessary measures are taken, if not by oneself then by an appropriate colleague.

The interpretative and supportive aspects of genetic counselling have been well outlined in a recent book written by a non-medical genetic counsellor[4]. Although the separation of diagnostic from counselling processes is not something that the author personally favours, the book clearly illustrates how easily the personal and social problems can be relegated by clinicians to a minor place, and how valuable repeated consultations, allowing a full discussion with the family, can be.

References
1. Porter I. H. (1977) *Evolution of Genetic Counseling in America*. In: Lubs H. A. and De La Cruz F. (ed.), *Genetic Counseling*. New York, Raven Press. pp. 17–34.
2. *International Directory of Genetic Services* (1977) National Foundation March of Dimes, New York.
3. Reed S. C. (1963) *Counselling in Medical Genetics*. Philadelphia, Saunders. 2nd ed.
4. Kelly P. (1977) *Dealing with Dilemma. A Manual for Genetic Counselors*. New York, Springer-Verlag.

Further Reading
A number of useful works are listed here that are relevant to the overall field of genetic counselling.

Introductory books on Medical Genetics
The reader has a choice of a number of excellent and relatively inexpensive books, approaching the subject from different angles.
Carter C. O. (1975) *An ABC of Medical Genetics*. London, Lancet.
Emery A. E. H. (1979) *Elements of Medical Genetics*. London, Churchill Livingstone.
Frazer Roberts J. and Pembrey M. (1978) *An Introduction to Medical Genetics*. London, Oxford University Press.
Thompson J. S. and Thompson M. W. (1980) *Genetics in Medicine*. Philadelphia, Saunders.

More general textbooks
Bodmer W. F. and Cavalli-Sforza L. L. (1976) *Genetics, Evolution, and Man*. Reading, Freeman.
Emery A. E. H. (1976) *Methodology in Medical Genetics*. London, Churchill Livingstone.

Genetic counselling
Fuhrmann W. and Vogel F. (1976) *Genetic Counseling: A Guide for the Practicing Physician*. Berlin, Springer-Verlag.
A concise and clearly written introduction on the subject.
Lubs H. A. and De La Cruz F. (ed.) (1977) *Genetic Counseling*. New York, Raven Press.
A symposium report containing some valuable chapters.
Murphy E. A. and Chase G. (1975) *Principles of Genetic Counseling*. Baltimore, Johns Hopkins University Press.
This valuable book takes a critical and rigorous theoretical approach. Do not be deterred by the mathematics!
Stevenson A. C., Davison B. C. and Oakes M. W. (1976) *Genetic Counselling*. Oxford, Blackwell.

Clinical 'workbench' books
Bergsma D. (ed.) (1979) *Birth Defects Atlas and Compendium*. Baltimore, Williams & Wilkins.
A useful source of information, but data on genetic risks often inaccurate.
McKusick V. A. (1978) *Mendelian Inheritance in Man*. Baltimore, Johns Hopkins University Press.
This unique and invaluable source-book is an essential companion for anyone working with genetic disorders.

Smith D. A. (1977) *Recognisable Patterns of Human Malformation*. Philadelphia,
    Saunders.
    A valuable guide to 'syndromes'.
The Clinical Delineation of Birth Defects. Vols. 1–16. Baltimore, Williams & Wilkins.
    A valuable series of volumes covering inherited disorders of the major systems
    with numerous detailed case reports.

CHAPTER TWO

Genetic Counselling in Mendelian Disorders

When assessing the clinical and genetic information available for a family with a particular disorder, the primary question requiring an answer is — does the disorder follow Mendelian inheritance? If the answer is 'yes', then it is likely that precise and well-established risks can be given regarding its occurrence in other family members; if the answer is 'no', then the information that can be given is usually much less certain, though fortunately the risks are also likely to be lower than for Mendelian inheritance. If, as is often the case, the answer is not clear, then the right initial course may be to attempt to obtain further evidence rather than to give risks which may require radical revision.

Mendelian inheritance may be established in several ways, and the more independent evidence one has supporting the same conclusion, the more confident one can be that the risks one has given are correct. In some cases, the pattern of transmission of the disorder in the family may be conclusive, even if the diagnosis is unknown, or proves to be erroneous. Thus the pedigrees shown in *Figs.* 2.1 and 2.2 could hardly be anything else than autosomal dominant and X-linked recessive respectively. Nevertheless, one can be mistaken even in what appears to be the classical pattern, as in *Fig.* 2.3, where an infective basis was shown for an apparently typical Mendelian pedigree.

More commonly, Mendelian inheritance is established by a combination of clinical diagnosis with a compatible, but not in itself conclusive, pedigree pattern. Thus the pedigree shown in *Fig.* 2.4 is suggestive of autosomal dominant inheritance but could be a chance concentration of cases of a non-Mendelian, or even non-genetic disorder. The knowledge that the diagnosis in the family was Huntington's chorea would remove all doubt and allow genetic counselling to be given accordingly.

Not infrequently the pedigree information is entirely unhelpful and one is completely dependent on the clinical diagnosis. Nowhere is this seen more clearly than in the 'sporadic case' as shown in *Fig.* 2.5, where there are the following possibilities:

1. The disorder is largely or entirely non-genetic, with insignificant recurrence risk.

2. The disorder is polygenic or chromosomal in basis, with a definite (usually low to moderate) recurrence risk depending on the disorder.

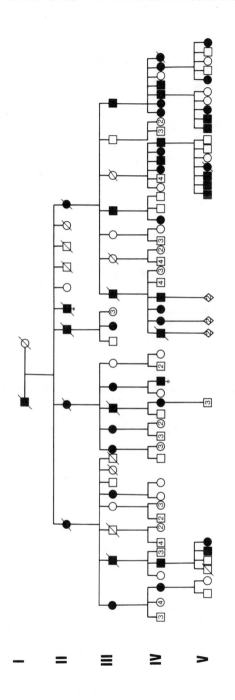

Fig. 2.1. Typical autosomal dominant inheritance (a South Wales kindred with Huntington's chorea). The disorder is transmitted by affected individuals to around half of their offspring. Both sexes transmit and develop the condition equally. The only unaffected individual to transmit the disorder died young and would presumably have developed it herself at a later date. (From Harper [3].)

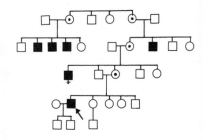

Fig. 2.2. Typical X-linked recessive inheritance. (A South Wales kindred with Becker (late onset X-linked) muscular dystrophy.) In each generation the disorder has been transmitted by healthy females, but only males are affected. The propositus has *not* transmitted the disorder to his sons.

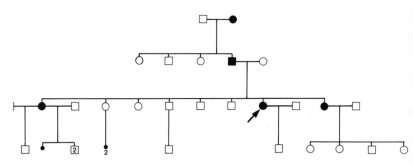

Fig. 2.3. Pedigree pattern mimicking autosomal dominant inheritance (familial Alzheimer's disease). Although the vertical transmission in this pedigree is extremely suggestive of autosomal dominant inheritance, a transmissible agent was isolated from the brain of the proposita.(From Harper[4] ; family reported by Gajdusek.)

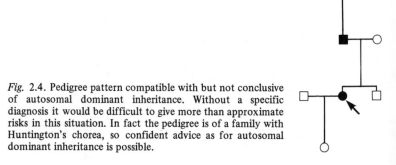

Fig. 2.4. Pedigree pattern compatible with but not conclusive of autosomal dominant inheritance. Without a specific diagnosis it would be difficult to give more than approximate risks in this situation. In fact the pedigree is of a family with Huntington's chorea, so confident advice as for autosomal dominant inheritance is possible.

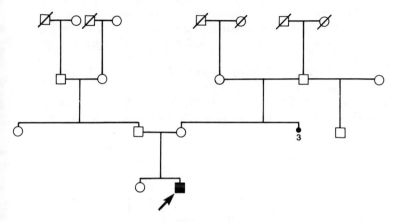

Fig. 2.5. A 'sporadic case' of a disorder – the commonest form of pedigree seen in genetic counselling. The affected individual could be the result of a non-genetic process, the family could represent autosomal dominant, autosomal recessive or X-linked inheritance, or a chromosomal or polygenic disorder. The absence of other affected family members does *not* mean that the disorder is not genetic.

3. Inheritance may be autosomal recessive, with a 1 in 4 recurrence risk to further children of either sex.

4. The disorder may represent a new dominant mutation, with negligible recurrence risk.

5. The disorder may be X-linked recessive, and the mother may or may not be a carrier.

Clearly the conclusion reached (if any) will depend on the accuracy of diagnosis and whether the disorder is known constantly to follow a mode of Mendelian inheritance. Thus if the diagnosis were classic achondroplasia, one could confidently predict the case represented a new dominant mutation, whereas with some complex and atypical malformation syndrome, no definite conclusion might be possible.

Although such an example may be regarded as extreme, reduction in family size means that the 'isolated case' is rapidly becoming the typical one for genetic counselling, a trend that will certainly continue. It is no more logical to await the occurrence of a classic pedigree pattern in a family than it is to delay the diagnosis of a disorder by waiting until the full clinical picture has developed.

Autosomal Dominant Inheritance

Although in theory this mode of inheritance is the simplest for genetic counselling, in practice it provides some of the most difficult problems, with some traps for the unwary that require special mention.

An autosomal dominant disorder or trait can be defined as one that is largely or completely expressed in the heterozygote. The homozygous state is either unknown or excessively rare in dominantly inherited disorders, but when it does occur is usually much more severe than the normal heterozygous form (e.g. familial hypercholesterolaemia), or lethal (e.g. achondroplasia).

In its fully developed form, the pattern of autosomal dominant inheritance is characteristic (*Fig.* 2.1) and allows precise risks to be given as illustrated in *Fig.* 2.6. The risk to offspring of affected members will be one-half, regardless of sex and regardless of whether the disease is fully

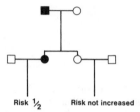

Fig. 2.6. Genetic risks in classic autosomal dominant inheritance.

developed or preclinical. The risk for offspring and more distant descendants of unaffected family members is not increased over the general population risk, provided that one can be sure that the individual really is unaffected.

Problems arise from the variability of gene expression that is seen in many dominantly inherited disorders and which may result from the influence of the normal allele that is also present.

1. *Late or Variable Onset*
This can be a major counselling problem, as in such disorders as Huntington's chorea and adult polycystic kidney disease. Here genetic counselling for an *affected* person provides no problems in risk estimation but the question, how old does one have to be before one is certain of *not* developing the disorder?, may be extremely difficult. The best approach is to use a 'life table' such as that for Huntington's chorea given on p. 138. Unfortunately, for most disorders there is either insufficient information or too much variation in families, while for some, such as myotonic dystrophy, the discrepancy between age at onset and first detection of the disease, may be extreme. More prospective data need to be collected to answer this question for late onset autosomal dominant disorders.

2. *Lack of Penetrance*
A small but important group of dominantly inherited disorders may show no evidence of disease in individuals known to possess the gene by reason of an affected parent and offspring. *Table* 2.1 lists some of these disorders, while *Fig.* 2.7 shows an example of lack of penetrance in hereditary

Table 2.1. Autosomal dominant disorders with lack of penetrance — some examples (penetrance estimates in brackets)

Hereditary pancreatitis (80%)
Gardner's syndrome (84%)
Retinoblastoma (80%)
Otosclerosis (40%)
Von Hippel—Lindau syndrome

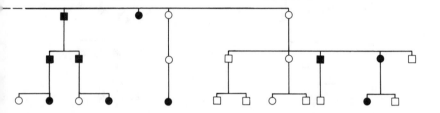

Fig. 2.7. Lack of penetrance in autosomal dominant inheritance. Part of a large kindred with hereditary pancreatitis. Three apparently normal individuals have transmitted the disorder to their descendants. (Adapted from Sibert, by permission of the author.)

pancreatitis. In part this is determined by how hard one looks for minor or subclinical signs, and what biochemical or other diagnostic tests are available. Thus careful biochemical study of family members in acute porphyrias will show some who are biochemically affected but have never had clinical features. Age is also a relevant factor; thus the gene for Huntington's chorea is 100 per cent penetrant at age of 70 but only about 50 per cent or so at age 40. Conversely, penetrance may decrease with age, as with petit mal epilepsy, where the proportion of family members that can be shown to be affected clinically or by EEG decreases after adolescence. Some disorders, of which retinoblastoma is the most notable, show lack of penetrance unrelated to age or to other detectable factors.

3. *Variation in Expression*
This refers to the degree to which the disorder is expressed in an individual, unlike penetrance, which is an index of the proportion of individuals with the gene showing it. Although some disorders (e.g. achondroplasia) are expressed with little variation, this is the exception rather than the rule for dominantly inherited disorders, so that it is wise never to assume a family member is unaffected without careful examination. In some disorders variability is so marked that special care is needed and radiological and other tests may be required; tuberous sclerosis and myotonic dystrophy are notable examples. Apparent inconsistencies such as 'skipped

generations' may be explained in this way (*Fig.* 2.8) and what is apparently
a new mutation may be shown to be a transmitted case (*Fig.* 2.9).

Variation in expression also produces another problem in genetic counselling. Because those individuals who reproduce tend to be the least
severely affected, the severity of a variable disorder is likely to be greater

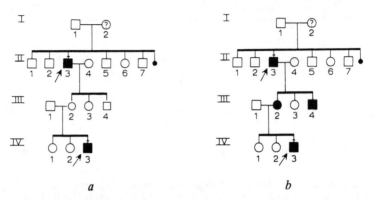

Fig. 2.8. Apparent 'skipped generation' in myotonic dystrophy. *a*, Pedigree before
investigation of generation III. *b*, Pedigree after full investigation. There is no skip-
ping of generations and the pattern of transmission is compatible with autosomal
dominant inheritance. (From Harper[6].)

in the child than in the parent and this must be made clear to potential
parents. Tuberous sclerosis provides a striking example of this. In addition,
one may have to consider the influence of the maternal intrauterine
environment, which appears to influence severity of expression in myotonic dystrophy and possibly in neurofibromatosis.

4. *Other Modifying Influences*

If variation in penetrance and expression reach more than a certain level it
becomes meaningless to consider the disorder as following Mendelian
inheritance. Nevertheless there are numerous influences which can modify
a basic autosomal dominant pattern, including sex (as in early male baldness)
drugs (as in the acute porphyrias) and diet (as in familial hypercholesterolaemia). The possibility of genetic heterogeneity must also be considered,
though at present there are few dominantly inherited disorders for which
this can be firmly established on either genetic or biochemical grounds.

5. *The New Mutation*

The dangers of assuming that an isolated case of a dominantly inherited
disorder represents a new mutation have already been mentioned. It is
important to establish this accurately since if it is, the risk of recurrence

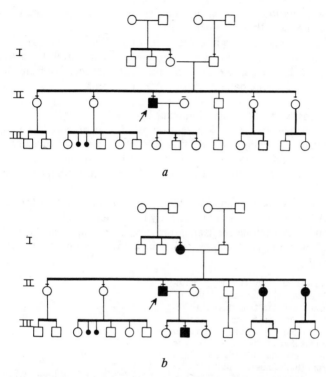

Fig. 2.9. Apparent new mutation in a family with myotonic dystrophy. *a*, Pedigree on initial investigation. The propositus appears to be the result of a new mutation. *b*, Pedigree after full investigation of asymptomatic members. (From Harper[6].)

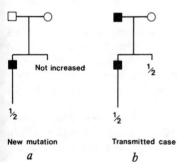

Fig. 2.10. Autosomal dominant inheritance. Genetic risks for new mutations and for transmitted case.

in a sib is no greater than for the general population (*Fig.* 2.10). The proportion of cases of a disorder resulting from new mutations will be directly related to the degree to which the disease interferes with reproduction, i.e. its genetic fitness. Thus, almost all cases of Apert's syndrome are new mutations, whereas in Huntington's chorea, the proportion is probably no more than 2–3 per cent.

It is important to recognize that a new mutation, once it has occurred, is permanent. Thus a patient representing a new mutation for achondroplasia (*Fig.* 2.10*a*) has the same 50 per cent chance of transmitting the condition as does the patient with an affected parent.

Homozygosity in Autosomal Dominant Disease

Almost all patients seen with autosomal dominant conditions will be heterozygotes, having inherited their disorder from only one side of the family or representing new mutations. Homozygosity requires both parents to have transmitted the gene, and this is most unlikely to happen unless either:

    a. The gene is common and relatively mild or late onset in its effects, or
    b. Affected individuals preferentially marry one another.

Familial hypercholesterolaemia provides an example of the first situation; the heterozygote frequency may be as high as 1 in 500, so one might

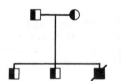

Fig. 2.11. Homozygosity for an autosomal dominant disorder achondroplasia. The parents and the two surviving children all have classic achondroplasia; they are represented by half shading to indicate that they are heterozygotes. The third child received the achondroplasia gene from both parents and had the lethal homozygous form, dying from respiratory insufficiency soon after birth. It can be seen that the pedigree is analogous to that commonly seen with autosomal recessive inheritance except that the heterozygotes are affected, not carriers.

expect chance marriages between such individuals to occur with a frequency of 1 in 250 000. Since only a quarter of the offspring of such a couple would be homozygous, one would expect the frequency of homozygotes only to be 1 in 1 million, and they are indeed exceedingly rare. Consanguinity would of course increase the chance of homozygosity, exactly as in autosomal recessive inheritance.

The situation more likely to be met in a genetic counselling clinic is where two individuals with the same disorder marry preferentially. This is seen not infrequently in achondroplasia (*Fig.* 2.11); the risks for the offspring in such a situation will be:

    one-quarter homozygous affected,
    one-half heterozygous achondroplastic,
    one-quarter unaffected.

In achondroplasia, the affected homozygote usually dies rapidly on

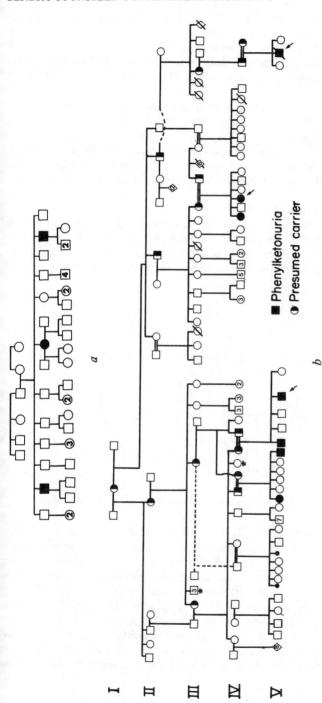

Phenylketonuria
Presumed carrier

Fig. 2.12. Patterns of autosomal recessive inheritance. Although many cases of autosomal recessive disease are isolated ones, a characteristic pedigree pattern is seen with large or inbred families. *a*, Limb girdle muscular dystrophy in a large South Wales sibship. Three out of 12 sibs are affected, including both sexes, but neither parent had muscle disease and the disorder has not been transmitted by the affected members or by their sibs. *b*, Phenylketonuria in an inbred Welsh Gypsy kindred. The affected individuals have been born to healthy but heterozygous parents in this highly inbred kindred. The gene can be traced back to a single ancestral heterozygote. (From Harper [3].)

account of the constricted chest; most other homozygotes known for dominant disorders are likewise very severe or lethal. Some (e.g. Huntington's chorea) have not been observed even though a number of marriages between heterozygotes are recorded; it is possible here that the homozygote may be spontaneously aborted, or (less likely) that it is indistinguishable from the heterozygote.

A somewhat similar (though rare) situation may occur when marriage partners have different, but allelic disorders. The child may then receive both abnormal alleles and will appear as a 'genetic compound'. This has been recorded with achondroplasia and the milder dysplasia hypochondroplasia. The resulting child was more severely affected than either parent, but less severely affected than the homozygote for achondroplasia.

Autosomal Recessive Inheritance

The principal difficulty with autosomal recessive inheritance is to be sure that this is indeed the mode of inheritance in a particular family. The great majority of cases of an autosomal recessive disorder are born to healthy but heterozygous parents, with no other affected relatives. Vertical

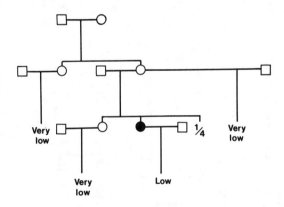

Fig. 2.13. Genetic risks in autosomal recessive inheritance.

transmission, so characteristic of dominant inheritance, is rarely seen (*Fig.* 2.12), and with the small families of the present time it is unusual to see more than one, or at most two affected sibs. Thus autosomal recessive disorders, even more than autosomal dominant, usually have to be detected from the isolated case, with little or no genetic information to help.

Where the diagnosis makes this mode of inheritance certain, or in the minority of families where the genetic pattern is clear, risk prediction is relatively simple (*Fig.* 2.13). In the great majority of instances the only significant increase in risk is for sibs of the affected individual, for whom the risk is 1/4. Unless the disorder is especially common or there is consanguinity, the risks for half sibs, children and in particular for children of healthy sibs is only minimally increased over that for the general population. The precise risk will depend on the frequency of heterozygotes in the population, since it will be necessary for both partners to contribute the abnormal gene for a child to be affected. It is thus important to know how to estimate the chance of being a carrier for an autosomal recessive disorder, both for family members and for the general population, and this is outlined below.

Risk of Being a Carrier

1. *Risk Within a Family (Fig. 2.14).* The parents and children of a patient with an autosomal recessive disorder are obligatory carriers, while second-degree relatives (uncles, aunts, nephews, nieces, half sibs, grandparents)

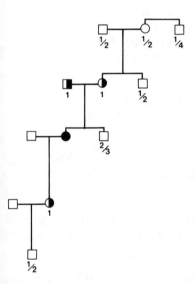

Fig. 2.14. Risks of being a carrier in autosomal recessive inheritance. (Obligatory carriers are half shaded.)

will have a chance of one-half of being a carrier. Each further step will reduce the risk by one-half, so that it is relatively simple to estimate the chance of any relative being a carrier if their closeness to the patient is known (*see also* p. 103). Sibs provide a special case: although the chance that the child of two carrier parents will itself be a carrier is 2 out of 4, the chance of a *healthy* sib being a carrier is 2 out of 3, since the affected category of individuals has been removed from consideration.

When calculating the risks for a family member being a carrier, the possibility of new mutation can be ignored since it is excessively rare in relation to the other risks. Likewise, although the general population risk must in theory be added, this is insignificant except for the commonest disorders.

2. *Population Risk.* It is rare for the population frequency of carriers for an autosomal recessive disease to be known by direct observation, but fortunately it can be estimated from the disease frequency by the relationship known as the Hardy—Weinberg equilibrium. In the few cases where direct observations are available, they agree closely with the predicted frequencies, so it seems reasonable to rely on them at least as an approximation.

The basis of the Hardy—Weinberg equilibrium and the possible reasons for variation from it are covered fully in genetics texts and are not given here. What the clinician needs to know is that the gene frequency and heterozygote frequency can be predicted, provided that the frequency of the affected homozygotes is known. For the usual situation where one has two alleles:

The commoner 'normal' allele with frequency p.

and the rarer 'disease' allele with frequency q.

(whose combined frequency must equal 1)

The proportions of the following categories are as follows:

q^2 Abnormal homozygotes (= disease frequency)

p^2 Normal homozygotes

2pq   Heterozygotes

The starting point is the disease frequency which is often known.

The square root of this gives the 'abnormal' gene frequency q.

From this one can obtain p which must be $1 - q$.

This allows one to work out the carrier frequency 2pq.

In practice p (the 'normal' gene frequency) is close to 1 except for exceedingly common diseases, so 2pq differs little from 2q

i.e. for rare recessive disorders, the carrier frequency is twice the square root of the disease frequency.

If the above over-simplification helps non-genetically-minded clinicians it will be more than worth any retribution the author receives from his fellow geneticists!

If we now return to our practical counselling situation, we can readily estimate the risk for offspring of patients with a recessively inherited disease and for their sibs and other relatives. *Table* 2.2 gives the risks for a range of gene frequencies. It can be seen that only for the commonest of recessive disorders do the risks become considerable, so that whether a relative is or is not a carrier is not of critical importance unless they are marrying a close relative. (*See also* Chapter 5.)

Consanguinity

The estimation of genetic risks in relation to consanguinity is discussed fully in Chapter 7, but needs a mention here in relation to autosomal recessive inheritance, since it is this category of disorders that is principally influenced by it. Several points need to be emphasized:

Table 2.2. Risks of transmitting an autosomal recessive disorder in relation to disease incidence (the spouse is assumed to be healthy and unrelated)

Disease frequency (per 10 000)	Gene frequency (%)	Carrier frequency (%)	Risk for offspring of affected homozygote (%)	Risk for offspring of healthy sib (%)
100	10·0	18·0	9·0	3·0
50	7·1	13·2	6·6	2·2
20	4·5	8·6	4·3	1·4
10	3·2	6·2	3·1	1·0
8	2·8	5·4	2·7	0·9
6	2·4	4·7	2·3	0·78
5	2·2	4·3	2·1	0·72
4	2·0	3·9	2·0	0·65
2	1·4	2·8	1·4	0·46
1	1·0	2·0	1·0	0·33
0·5	0·71	1·4	0·70	0·23
0·1	0·32	0·64	0·32	0·11
0·05	0·22	0·44	0·22	0·07
0·01	0·10	0·20	0·10	0·03

1. Consanguinity is only relevant to genetic risks if it involves *both* parental lines, not just one, as shown below:

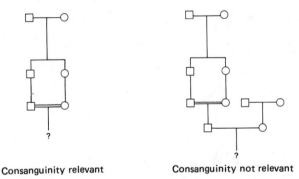

Consanguinity relevant   Consanguinity not relevant

2. Two brothers marrying two sisters (or similar combinations) as shown below do *not* constitute consanguinity.

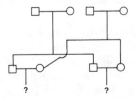

3. The rarer the disorder, the higher will be the proportion of affected individuals resulting from consanguineous marriages.

4. The presence of consanguinity in relation to a syndrome of uncertain inheritance favours, but does not prove autosomal recessive inheritance.

5. Consanguinity must be seen in the context of the particular community – thus in a population where 30 per cent of marriages are between cousins, an apparent relationship of a particular disorder with consanguinity is much less certain than in a population where there is only 1 per cent of cousin marriages.

6. Extensive consanguinity can give the appearance of autosomal dominant inheritance, with vertical transmission resulting from an affected person marrying a carrier, as shown in *Fig. 2.15.*

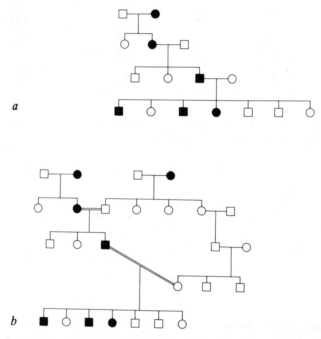

Fig. 2.15. *a,* An incomplete pedigree showing quasi-dominant inheritance of alkaptonuria. *b,* The complete pedigree showing that consanguinity accounts for the pedigree pattern simulating autosomal dominant inheritance. (After Khachadurian A. K. and Feisal K. A. *J. Chronic Dis.* 7 (1958) 455 and McKusick (1969)).

Other Problems with Autosomal Recessive Disease
Once one is confident that this is indeed the mode of inheritance, the difficulties in genetic counselling are much less than those encountered in autosomal dominant disorders. In particular, lack of penetrance is rarely encountered and variation in expression is much less. Genetic hetero-

geneity is probably the major cause of variation within an apparently single entity; sometimes this can be recognized biochemically, as in many of the inborn errors of metabolism; in other conditions it must be inferred from family data. An example of the practical importance of recognizing such heterogeneity is seen in the different types of recessively inherited polycystic kidney disease in which sibs show close concordance in age of onset and death (*see* Chapter 18); a corresponding situation is seen in the spinal muscular atrophies (*see* Chapter 9) where the classic Werdnig— Hoffman disease shows close similarity between sibs whereas the later onset form shows a much broader scatter. Information of this type on the likely prognosis is just as important for parents contemplating another pregnancy as is the actual risk of recurrence.

A further factor of particular relevance for autosomal recessive disorders is the availability of prenatal diagnosis in many cases, especially those where the underlying biochemical defect is known. This is discussed in Chapter 6. The use of AID (artificial insemination by donor) is also relevant in recessive disorders, since the risk of an unrelated donor being a carrier for the same gene is small.

A final factor, again related to the fact that an autosomal recessive disorder necessitates both parents being carriers, is the outlook for parents remarrying. With the frequency of divorce at its current level in most of Europe and America, this must be a serious consideration when sterilization is being considered in either parent. It is, however, a difficult subject even to discuss with parents, particularly when the burden of an affected child is likely to be a major factor in the break-up of a marriage.

Conversely the necessary contribution of both parents to an autosomal recessive disorder in a child can be a positive feature in genetic counselling. It is frequently found that one parent (commonly the mother) is assuming the burden of guilt for the occurrence of the disorder, and this may be reinforced by the views (spoken or tacit) of other relatives. The realization that 'one side of the family' is not to blame, and that everyone carries at least one harmful genetic factor, is frequently a great relief to couples to whom a child with an autosomal recessive disorder has been born.

Marriages Between Two Affected Individuals

This situation has already been discussed for autosomal dominant disorders, and is seen rather more frequently with those showing autosomal recessive inheritance. The usual reason is preferential marriage between similarly affected people, particularly those with blindness or deafness, who may be educated together and have a common social bond. Albinism and severe congenital deafness provide the two best documented examples.

If two individuals with the same disorder marry (e.g. the severe form of oculocutaneous albinism), all offspring must be affected, since each parent can only transmit an abnormal gene (a) as shown below.

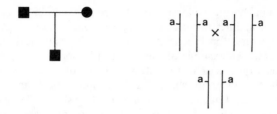

It is crucial, however, to be sure that genetic heterogeneity does not exist, since if the parents' disorders are controlled by different loci, all offspring will be *unaffected*, though carriers at both loci; a greater potential for erroneous counselling cannot be imagined!

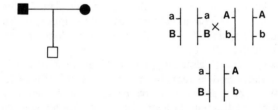

In the case of albinism careful study will usually distinguish the two forms (*see* Chapter 14). In severe congenital deafness, however, this is impossible, so that advice must be based on knowledge of the number and relative frequency of the different types, and on whether the couple concerned have already had affected or normal children. This situation is one of the many in genetic counselling where the recognition of genetic heterogeneity is of extreme importance.

X-linked Disease

Since no serious human diseases are known to be borne on the Y chromosome sex-linkage is equivalent to X-linkage, so far as genetic counselling is concerned. X-linkage produces some unusual problems which are of considerable practical importance, and as a result X-linked disorders occupy a much more prominent place in a genetic counselling clinic than would be expected from the relative contribution of the X chromosome to the human genome.

Over 100 definitely X-linked human disorders or traits have been recognized, and as complete a list of disorders as possible is given in *Table* 2.3. It can be seen that the great majority are classed as X-linked recessive, with a much smaller number as dominant and a few as dominant but lethal in the hemizygous male. The terms 'dominant' and 'recessive' must be used with caution in X-linked disease, since a much greater degree of

Table 2.3. Mendelian disorders following X-linked inheritance (after McKusick, 1978)

Addison's disease with cerebral sclerosis	Hypophosphataemic rickets
Adrenal hypoplasia (one type)	Icthyosis (steroid sulphatase deficiency)
Agammaglobulinaemia, Bruton type (sometimes also Swiss type)	Incontinentia pigmenti
	Kallmann's syndrome
Albinism, ocular	Keratosis follicularis spinulosa
Albinism–deafness syndrome	Lesch–Nyhan syndrome (hypoxanthine-guanine-phosphoribosyl transferase deficiency)
Aldrich's syndrome	
Alport's syndrome (some kindreds)	
Amelogenesis imperfecta (two types)	
Anaemia, hereditary hypochromic	Lowe (oculocerebrorenal) syndrome
Angiokeratoma (Fabry's disease)	Macular dystrophy of the retina (one type)
Cataract, congenital (one type)	
Cerebellar ataxia (one type)	Menkes syndrome
Cerebral sclerosis, diffuse	Mental retardation, Renpenning type
Charcot–Marie–Tooth peroneal muscular atrophy (one type)	Microphthalmia with multiple anomalies (Lenz syndrome)
Choroideraemia	Mucopolysaccharidosis II (Hunter's syndrome)
Choroidoretinal degeneration (one rare type)	Muscular dystrophy, Becker, Duchenne and Dreifuss types
Coffin–Lowry syndrome	Myotubular myopathy (one type)
Colour blindness (several types)	Night blindness, congenital stationary
Deafness, perceptive (several types)	Norrie's disease (pseudoglioma)
Diabetes insipidus, nephrogenic	Nystagmus, oculomotor or 'jerky'
Diabetes insipidus, neurohypophyseal (some families)	Ornithine transcarbamylase deficiency (Type I hyperammonaemia)
Dyskeratosis congenita	Orofaciodigital syndrome
Ectodermal dysplasia, anhidrotic	Phosphoglycerate kinase deficiency
Ehlers–Danlos syndrome, type V	Phosphoribosylpyrophosphate (PRPP) synthetase deficiency
Faciogenital dysplasia (Aarskog's syndrome)	Reifenstein's syndrome
Focal dermal hypoplasia	Retinitis pigmentosa (one type)
Glucose-6-phosphate dehydrogenase deficiency	Retinoschisis
	Spastic paraplegia (one type)
Glycogen storage disease, type VIII	Spinal muscular atrophy (one type)
Gonadal dysgenesis (XY female type)	Spondylo-epiphyseal dysplasia tarda
Granulomatous disease (NADPH oxidase deficiency)	Testicular feminization syndrome
	Thrombocytopenia, hereditary (one type)
Haemophilia A	
Haemophilia B	Thyroxine-binding globulin absence or variants of
Hydrocephalus (aqueduct stenosis, one type)	Xg blood group system

variability in the heterozygous female is seen than is the case with autosomal disorders. This is largely the result of X-chromosome inactivation (the Lyon hypothesis), which appears to affect almost the entire X-chromosome in the human female. One of the two X-chromosomes is randomly inactivated in early embryonic life and becomes visible as the 'sex chromatin' or 'Barr' body under the nuclear membrane. Since the descendants of each cell retain the same inactivated X-chromosome it follows that a female heterozygous for an X-linked disorder or trait will be a mosaic, with two populations of cells, one of which has the 'normal', the other the 'abnormal' X-chromosome functioning.

There is a considerable amount of direct evidence for X-chromosome inactivation in human diseases, which may be expressed in several ways. Some disorders show 'patchy' changes in heterozygotes; thus patchy retinal changes are seen in carriers for X-linked retinitis pigmentosa and choroideraemia, and patchy muscle biopsy changes may be found in carriers for Duchenne muscular dystrophy. More commonly, variability in X-inactivation is seen in a milder and more variable expression of clinical and biochemical changes. Thus in X-linked hypophosphataemic rickets, generally considered to be an X-linked dominant, affected females have milder or even subclinical disease; conversely in haemophilia, usually classed as an X-linked recessive, some carriers show a mild bleeding tendency in addition to reduced levels of Factor VIII. The implications for tests of carrier detection in X-linked diseases are discussed in Chapter 5.

The Recognition of X-linkage

Recognition of an X-linked pedigree pattern is crucial to correct genetic counselling and is surprisingly often overlooked. The following criteria apply regardless of whether the disorder is recessive, dominant or intermediate in expression. *Figs.* 2.16–2.21 give some examples.

1. Male to male transmission *never* occurs, since a man never hands his X chromosome to his son.

2. All daughters of an affected male will receive the gene, i.e. they will all be affected if the inheritance is X-linked dominant, all carriers if it is X-linked recessive.

3. Unaffected males never transmit the disease to descendants of either sex.

4. The risk to sons of women who are definite carriers (or affected in the case of an X-linked dominant) is one-half.

5. Half the daughters of carrier women will themselves be carriers. In the case of an X-linked dominant half the daughters of affected women will be affected.

6. Affected homozygous females are exceptional in X-linked recessive disorders, and will only occur when an affected male marries a carrier female; in X-linked dominant inheritance twice as many females will on average be affected as males.

These simple guidelines will cover most genetic counselling problems and will allow a definite decision to be made in most instances as to whether the disorder is X-linked or not. It can be seen that the situation is essentially similar for X-linked recessive and X-linked dominants, the heterozygous women in the latter group being affected rather than carriers. Apparent anomalies may be the result of chromosome disorders (e.g. occurrence of the disease in a 45 X 0 female (*see Fig.* 2.21)) or to non-paternity. Some particular problems are shown below.

1. The classic X-linked recessive pattern. *Fig.* 2.16 shows this in a family with haemophilia A.

2. Disorders where affected males do not reproduce (*Fig.* 2.17). This may result from the severity of the disease (e.g. Duchenne muscular

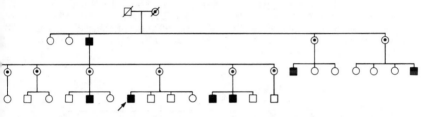

Fig. 2.16. Typical X-linked recessive inheritance (haemophilia A). Note that *all* sons of an affected male are healthy, while all daughters are carriers. The disorder is transmitted by healthy females and is confined to males, but these features are less critical than the lack of male to male transmission in establishing or disproving X-linkage.

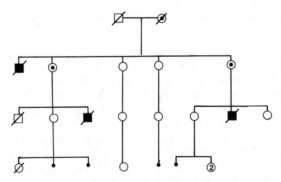

Fig. 2.17. Presumed X-linked inheritance. Duchenne muscular dystrophy in a South Wales kindred. Although the disorder is confined to males and is transmitted by healthy females as expected with X-linked recessive inheritance, the lack of reproduction by affected males means that the critical test of lack of male to male transmission cannot be seen.

dystrophy) or from infertility (e.g. Kallmann's syndrome). Here the test of male to male transmission cannot be applied, so unless one has other genetic data (e.g. linkage markers or occurrence in an X 0 female) X-linkage is presumed rather than proven.

3. X-linked dominant inheritance (*Fig.* 2.18). The pattern may at first glance be mistaken for autosomal dominant inheritance, but if offspring of

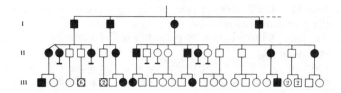

Fig. 2.18. X-linked dominant inheritance in a family with familial hypophosphataemia (vitamin D resistant rickets). (*After* McKusick.) The pattern is superficially similar to autosomal dominant inheritance but when the offspring of affected males are considered it becomes clear that all daughters are affected, but that the disorder is never transmitted from father to son.

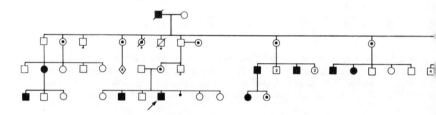

Fig. 2.19. Intermediate X-linked inheritance. A South Wales kindred with hereditary oculomotor nystagmus. The pattern is recognized by examining the offspring of affected males. All sons are unaffected, but all daughters are either affected or prove to be carriers.

affected males are considered, all sons are unaffected, all daughters are affected. The excess of affected females can also be seen.

4. 'Intermediate' X-linked inheritance. The blurred distinction between dominant and recessive in X-linked disease has already been mentioned. In a few conditions heterozygotes may show the disease in one branch of a family, but not in another. *Fig.* 2.19 shows an example of this. Although at first sight the pattern appears confusing, the situation is soon clarified if the offspring of affected males are considered – all sons are unaffected while the females are either affected or carriers.

5. X-linked dominant inheritance with lethality in the male. Here the disorder is only seen in the heterozygous females, the affected (hemizygous) males being undetected or appearing as an excess of spontaneous abortions. It is difficult to prove this situation, but it is strongly suspected for several disorders, including focal dermal hypoplasia and incontentia pigmenti. Genetic counselling requires some care; leaving aside spontaneous abortions, one-third of the offspring of an affected woman will be affected; all the liveborn males will be unaffected, as will half of the females. Two-thirds of all children will be female. Fetal sexing with termination of female pregnancies may be considered. Where an affected child has been born to healthy parents this is likely to represent a new mutation and the

recurrence risk is likely to be low (though no satisfactory data exist on this point).

6. Common X-linked genes. Where an X-linked gene is common in a particular population, confusing pedigree patterns may be produced. This may be seen with colour-blindness in European populations and with G6PD deficiency in the Middle East. The marriage of affected males to heterozygous females is not infrequent and will result in homozygous females (*Fig.* 2.20), all of whose sons will be affected. A similar pattern can occasionally be seen with rarer disorders when there is consanguinity.

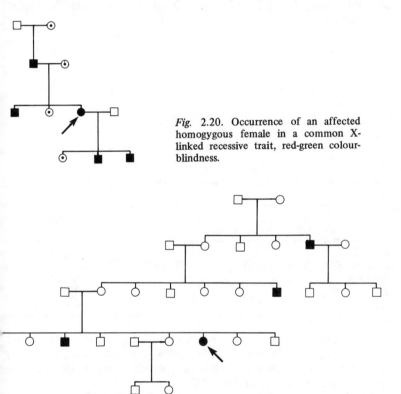

Fig. 2.20. Occurrence of an affected homogygous female in a common X-linked recessive trait, red-green colour-blindness.

Fig. 2.21. Where an affected girl is found to have a rare and clearly X-linked disorder, a sex chromosome abnormality such as the Turner (XO) syndrome should be considered. This proved to be the case in this family with X-linked cerebellar ataxia studied by Shokeir[7].

The Risk of Being a Carrier for an X-linked Disorder

Methods of carrier detection in X-linked disorders are discussed in Chapter 5, but it is clearly important to estimate the genetic risk of a female relative being a carrier so that information from carrier testing (if any) can be appropriately combined. The estimation of these risks is not always easy and is one of the few situations where a mathematical approach is needed in genetic counselling.

The clinician need not feel faint-hearted at the prospect of this, for it is likely that the majority of his geneticist colleagues will be as ignorant as himself! A recent questionnaire[1] sent to clinical geneticists in Britain concerning the estimation of carrier risks in Duchenne muscular dystrophy showed only a minority giving a completely correct reply to the questions. Leaving aside the problem of new mutations the situation can be approached as follows, using *Fig.* 2.22, a family with Duchenne muscular dystrophy, as an example.

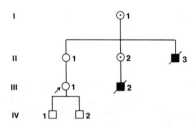

Fig. 2.22

Table 2.4. A working table to combine risk information for the pedigree shown in *Fig.* 2.22

	Consultand a carrier	Consultand not a carrier
Prior risk	1/4	3/4
Conditional risk (2 normal sons)	1/2 × 1/2 (= 1/4)	1
Joint risk	1/16	3/4 (= 12/16)
Relative risk	1	12
Final risk	1/13	12/13

1. Obligatory carriers should be identified — these are I — 1 and II — 2

2. The prior genetic risk of the individual requiring advice, sometimes referred to as the 'consultand' (arrowed) should be estimated. Here it is 1/4, since her mother's prior risk is 1/2.

3. Other relevant information must be incorporated. Here the relevant fact is that the consultand has had two normal sons (commonsense tells us that this makes it less likely that she is a carrier. The question is — how much less likely? In fact it can be estimated and combined with other information simply (using what is sometimes termed Bayes' theorem) by multiplying it with the corresponding prior risk. This is best done by constructing a table, which gives the chances of the two possibilities, shown in *Table* 2.4.

The prior risks are clearly 1/4 and 3/4 respectively.

The 'conditional' information resulting from the normal sons will give a chance of 1/2 for this happening once if she is a carrier and $1/2 \times 1/2 = 1/4$ for both sons being normal if she is a carrier (3 sons would give a risk of 1/8 and so on). The corresponding chance of 2 sons being normal if she is *not* a carrier is clearly 1 (100 per cent). The joint risk is then obtained by multiplying the two columns, and if they are placed over the same denominator (giving 1/16 and 12/16), the relative risk can be seen to be 1 *to* 12 that the consultand is a carrier, or a final risk of 1 in 13.

Care must be taken to relate the 'conditional' information to the correct person. Thus in *Fig.* 2.23, another Duchenne family, the normal

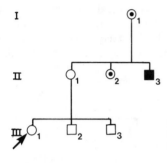

Fig. 2.23. Carrier risks with an X-linked recessive disorder (Duchenne muscular dystrophy.)

Table 2.5. Risks for II − 1

	Carrier	Not a carrier
Prior risk	1/2	1/2
Conditional risk	$1/2 \times 1/2$ (= 1/4)	1
Joint risk	1/8	1/2 (= 4/8)
Relative risks	1	4
Final risk	1/5	4/5
Prior risk for III − 1	1/10	

sons affect the chances of the *mother* of the consultand (II − 1) being a carrier, and the risk must be worked out for her before proceeding to the daughter (III − 1), whose prior risk (1/10) is half her mother's final risk (1/5) (*Table* 2.5). If the daughter herself had normal sons one could proceed as in the previous example but using the new prior risk of 1/10 as the starting point.

It can be seen that the use of genetic information in this way can substantially affect the risks given in genetic counselling and in general with a methodical approach the estimations are not difficult. Incorporation of data from more distant relationships can become complex but rarely affects the risks to a great extent. It is important to recognize that not only genetic information may be used in this way, but also data on carrier detection, such as may be available in haemophilia and Duchenne muscular dystrophy. Some examples of this are given in Chapter 6.

A final caution should be given; since all these estimates are based on uncertainty, they may need to be modified in the light of future events. Thus the birth of an affected child to II − 1 in *Fig.* 2.23 would make her an obligatory carrier and all previous estimates would have to be discarded in the light of this.

The Isolated Case of an X-linked Disorder
In autosomal dominant inheritance new mutations can usually be clearly distinguished from transmitted cases; in autosomal recessive disorders mutation plays an insignificant part in relation to transmitted genes and can be ignored in genetic counselling. In X-linked recessive disorders, however, it may be extremely difficult, if not impossible, to tell whether

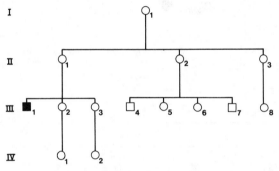

Fig. 2.24. An isolated case of a lethal X-linked disorder (Duchenne) muscular dystrophy. Is this a new mutation or not? *See* text and following figures for the estimation of carrier risks in this difficult situation.

an isolated case represents a new mutation or whether the mother is a carrier. Since an accurate distinction is essential for correct genetic counselling this situation needs careful consideration.

Where reliable methods of carrier detection exist, these should obviously be employed. Unfortunately, the variability of gene expression in hetero-zygotes for X-linked disease makes carrier detection difficult in a propor-tion of women even when tests exist. This is clearly seen in haemophilia A and Duchenne muscular dystrophy, where 20−30 per cent of known carriers show results of carrier tests falling within normal limits (*see* Chapter 5).

The example shown in *Fig.* 2.24 shows the practical aspect of the problem. Three possibilities exist to explain the occurrence of this isolated case of Duchenne muscular dystrophy.

1. III − 1 is the result of a new mutation. In this case none of the numerous female relatives is at significant risk of being a carrier.

2. The mother II − 1 is a carrier, but is herself the result of a new mutation. In this case, the daughters III − 2 and III − 3 are at 50 per cent risk of being carriers and their daughters IV − 1 and IV − 2 have a risk of 1/4. However, none of the other female relatives are at risk.

3. The disorder has been transmitted through the mother from the grandmother I − 1, in which case, in addition to those already mentioned as being at risk, II − 2 and II − 3 are at 50 per cent prior risk, with a risk of 1/4 for their daughters III − 5, 6 and 8.

Unfortunately, these three situations cannot always be distinguished with certainty by carrier testing, so a dilemma exists − should one reassure the numerous female relatives and risk an affected child being born to one of them, or should they be assumed to be carriers and advised to have fetal sexing in any pregnancies, in which case large numbers of healthy male fetuses might be needlessly aborted? The logical course is neither of these, but to attempt to work out the risk for the various family members as accurately as possible and to make further decisions in the light of this. The problem can be approached as follows:

1. The *prior* risk of II − 1 and I − 1 being carriers as opposed to III − 1 resulting from a new mutation must be estimated. From this the prior risk of other family members such as II − 2 and II − 3 can be estimated.

2. *Conditional* information (from normal sons and carrier testing results) can be tabulated as shown in the previous examples.

3. These pieces of information can be combined to give a final risk as already shown.

The difficult problem is to decide what is the *prior* risk that this isolated case has resulted from mutation or has been transmitted. It has long been assumed that for an isolated case of an X-linked recessive disorder in which affected males do not reproduce the proportions are as follows:

New mutation	Mother *not* carrier	1/3
Transmitted case	Mother carrier but *not* grandmother	1/3
Transmitted case	Mother and grandmother carriers	1/3

The derivation of this will not be given here, but using this information one can readily assign risks to the various women in the family as shown in *Fig. 2.25*. In *Fig. 2.25b* the information from the normal sons of II − 3 has also been incorporated, and it can be seen that the risks for III − 5 and III − 6 have been considerably lowered by the normal brothers. Carrier testing results would have produced further information which has been omitted for simplicity.

Unfortunately, there is considerable uncertainty as to whether the formula given above is generally applicable; it assumes equal mutation rates in the sexes, and it is possible, though not yet certain that in some disorders a higher proportion of mothers of isolated cases are carriers than

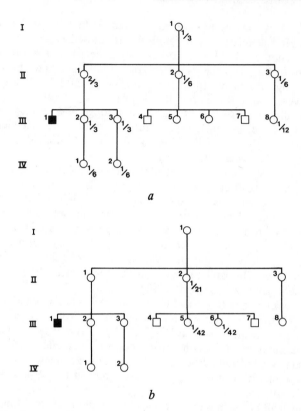

Fig. 2.25. *a,* Carrier risks for women in a family with a lethal X-linked disorder (Duchenne dystrophy) shown in *Fig.* 2.24 assuming 1/3 of cases due to new mutation. *b,* The same pedigree as in (*a*) showing the modification of risks from the normal sons of II-2.

the two-thirds expected. Certainly for disorders where the affected males reproduce, such as haemophilia and Becker muscular dystrophy, the proportion of carrier mothers of isolated cases is higher, and in the absence of other information it is wise to assume that such a woman is a carrier rather than the reverse. For Duchenne dystrophy most evidence favours the proportion of new mutations being close to the predicted 1/3 [2, 5].

References

1. Bundey S. E. (1978) Calculation of genetic risks in Duchenne muscular dystrophy by geneticists in the United Kingdom. *J. Med. Genet.* **15,** 249–253.
2. Davie A. M. and Emery A. E. H. (1978) Estimation of proportion of new mutants among cases of Duchenne muscular dystrophy. *J. Med. Genet.* **15,** 339–345.
3. Harper P. S. (1976) Genetic variation in Wales. *J. R. Coll. Physicians Lond.* **10,** 321–332.

4. Harper P. S. (1977) Mendelian inheritance or transmissible agent — the lesson of Kuru and the Australia Antigen. *J. Med. Genet.* **14**, 389–398.

5. Sibert J. R., Harper P. S., Thomson R. J. et al. (1979) Carrier detection in Duchenne muscular dystrophy. Evidence from a study of obligatory carriers and mothers of isolated cases. *Arch. Dis. Child.* **54**, 534–537.

6. Harper P. S. (1979) *Myotonic Dystrophy.* Philadelphia, Saunders.

7. Shokeir M. H. K. (1970) X-linked cerebellar ataxia. *Clin. Genet.* **1**, 225–231.

CHAPTER THREE

Genetic Counselling in non-Mendelian Disorders

A large group of disorders exists in which there appears to be a considerable genetic component but which follows no clear pattern of Mendelian inheritance and shows no identifiable abnormality in chromosome morphology. The terms 'polygenic' and 'multifactorial' inheritance have been used to cover this group, but in reality there is no single category that is satisfactory. In some instances, e.g. diabetes mellitus, one is dealing with a heterogeneous mixture of disorders, a few of which may be Mendelian, some largely environmental but at present not clearly distinguishable. In other cases, such as some of the congenital malformation sydromes, unidentified teratogens may be a contributing factor. In most instances, the disorder appears to result from the additive effect of a number of influences, some genetic, others environmental or unknown.

Whatever the theoretical basis of these disorders may be, they provide a large number of serious genetic counselling problems. Most of the commoner birth defects are non-Mendelian, as are most of the major chronic diseases of later life. In most cases one can give genetic advice which is reasonably accurate, even though it lacks the precision that is possible for disorders following Mendelian inheritance.

Empiric Risk Data

This impressive sounding term is merely a statement of the fact that someone has actually looked at what happens in a particular situation. Data on the risks to relatives are now available for a large number of non-Mendelian disorders and, provided the study has been careful and as far as possible unbiased, such information provides the most satisfactory basis for counselling. It has to be remembered, however, as stated in Chapter 1, that such risk figures are not universal in their application as are Mendelian ratios. In particular:

1. Data collected on one population may not be applicable to others where the incidence, and perhaps aetiology, of the disorder are different.

2. Improved classification of disorders, in particular resolution of heterogeneity or identification of specific causative factors, may require radical revision of risk estimates.

3. Risks may depend not only on the diagnosis but on individual factors such as sex, severity of disease and number of affected family members.

Empiric risk figures are given for as many disorders as possible in the specific sections of this book. The aspects to be discussed here are more general ones which will influence how these risk figures are applied and will also allow estimation of risks when no data derived from direct experience are available.

The Basis of 'Multifactorial' Inheritance

The essential distinguishing factor from the Mendelian disorders is that a single genetic locus cannot be held responsible for the condition and that

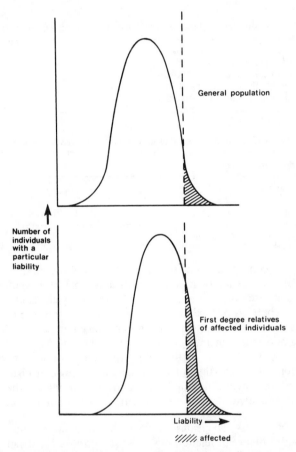

Fig. 3.1. Liability and genetic risks in multifactorial inheritance. The distribution of liability to the disorder in the general population follows an approximately 'normal' distribution, with individuals exceeding a certain threshold value being affected. First-degree relatives have a similar normal distribution of liability, but the curve is shifted to the right by the increased genetic component, so a greater proportion will exceed the threshold and be affected.

it is the result of the additive effect of a number of genetic loci and of a number of external factors. The sum of these determines a person's liability to be affected with the particular disorder, and this liability is expected to show a more or less 'normal' distribution in the population, with most people having an intermediate degree of liability and smaller numbers at each end of the distribution curve having unusually low or unusually high liability (*Fig.* 3.1). The last group form those who are actually affected, whose liability is above a postulated 'threshold' for the disorder.

Table 3.1. Multifactorial inheritance. Factors increasing risk to relatives

Close relationship to proband
High heritability of disorder
Proband of more rarely affected sex
Severe disease in proband
Multiple family members affected

Table 3.2. Recurrence risk of neural tube defects for different categories of relative

Relationship to proband	Risk
First degree (sibs)	5%
Second degree (nephews, nieces)	2%
Third degree (first cousins)	1% (or less)

(*See* Chapter 10 for full details.)

From this concept it can be seen that even a person with unusually high genetic liability may not be affected if environmental factors are favourable, and the converse will also apply. The degree to which liability is determined by genetic as opposed to environmental factors is often referred to as the *heritability* of a disorder, though in practice familial but non-genetic factors may often be included in this. The liability of relatives of a patient with the disorder will also be normally distributed in a similar way to the general population but the curve will be shifted towards higher liability because of the increased genetic component. Turning to the practical aspects, the following points are relevant; they are summarized in *Table* 3.1.

1. Increased risk is greatest among closest relatives and decreases rapidly with distance of relationship. It is rare to find a significant increase in risk for relatives more distant than second degree; even here risks are usually small. *Table* 3.2 shows the situation for neural tube defects.

2. The risk of recurrence will depend on the incidence of the disorder — unlike Mendelian inheritance. A useful approximation where specific figures are not available is that the maximum risk to first-degree relatives

is approximately the square root of the incidence, i.e. where the incidence is 1 in 10 000, the recurrence risk would be 1 in 100. The example of two congenital heart defects shown below, one common, the other relatively rare, shows the importance of this for counselling, since the recurrence risk for the commoner condition is three times that of the rarer.

Disorder	Approximate incidence (per 1000 live births)	Risk to sibs (%)
Ventricular septal defect	2	3
Common truncus arteriosus	0·15	1

3. Dominance and recessiveness do not generally apply. Thus the risk to sibs is comparable to that for children. Risks for offspring are not yet available for many birth defects, but can usually be taken as approximately equivalent to the risks for sibs in the absence of further information.

4. Where there is an unequal sex incidence, the risk is higher for relatives of a patient of the rarer sex; e.g. in pyloric stenosis, the risk for brothers of a male index case is 3·8 per cent but for brothers of a female index case 9·2 per cent (see Chapter 17). At first sight, this may seem unexpected, but when it is considered that girls require a greater genetic liability to develop the disorder than do boys, it can readily be seen that relatives of an affected girl will also have a greater genetic liability than where the index case is a boy.

5. The risk may be greater when the disorder is more severe. This is well shown in Hirschsprung's disease, where the risk for sibs of patients with long segment disease is greater than for those with a short segment affected (see Chapter 17). Again the greater severity reflects greater liability, part of which will be genetic and thus shared with relatives.

6. The risk is increased when multiple family members are affected. This is most clearly seen for neural tube defects, where the birth of a second affected sib increases the risk from 1 in 20 to 1 in 8 in a high-risk area such as S. Wales. This again results from the concentration of genetic liability in the particular family and is in contrast to the Mendelian situation where the number of affected family members (leaving aside mutation) is irrelevant. The influence of more distant relatives is less easy to determine, though computer programs have been developed to coordinate the information[1]. In general, one close (first-degree) relative outweighs numerous distant ones.

General Risks in non-Mendelian Disorders

There are many disorders for which adequate empiric risk figures do not yet exist. This may be because of rarity, or because the disorder is not sufficiently genetic in its determination for investigators to have found it worthwhile collecting such data. Often, there will be some evidence suggesting that genetic factors are involved, but it may not have been collected in a way that makes it suitable for giving genetic risks. Nevertheless, patients and relatives commonly enquire about risks, and it is helpful to be able to make an approximate estimate.

A variety of theoretical models of polygenic inheritance have been produced from which it is possible to work out risks to relatives[2]. Fortunately for the clinician, they arrive at broadly similar conclusions, so he need not be too concerned if he cannot understand the mathematics underlying them. This general agreement also suggests that they are likely to be reasonably correct. *Table* 3.3 summarizes some risk data of this type,

Table 3.3. Recurrence risks in multifactorial inheritance (based on Smith, 1971)

Population frequency %	Heritability %	Affected parents								
		0			1			2		
		Affected sibs								
		0	1	2	0	1	2	0	1	2
	80	1·0	6·5	14·2	8·3	18·5	27·8	40·9	46·6	51·6
1	50	1·0	3·9	8·4	4·3	9·3	15·1	14·6	20·6	26·3
	20	1·0	2·0	3·3	2·0	3·3	4·8	3·7	5·3	7·1
	80	0·1	2·5	8·2	2·9	9·8	17·9	31·7	37·4	42·4
0·1	50	0·1	1·0	3·2	1·0	3·4	6·9	6·6	10·9	15·3
	20	0·1	0·3	0·7	0·3	0·7	1·3	0·8	1·4	2·3

Extra data kindly provided by Dr Charles Smith and Dr Susan Holloway, Edinburgh.

based on the work of Smith[3] with some extra information kindly supplied. It can be seen that one needs to know several basic facts.

1. The frequency of the disorder. Figures are given here for a common disorder (1 per cent) e.g. a common cancer, and for a moderately frequent disorder (0·1 per cent).

2. Heritability. It should be possible to decide whether the disorder concerned is of high, moderate or low heritability, even though precise figures will rarely be available. Thus a common cancer would fall into the last group, whereas congenital heart disease would mostly be of high heritability.

3. Types of affected relative. Combinations of 0, 1 or 2 affected sibs and 0, 1 or 2 affected parents are given.

Clearly a table such as this cannot cover all situations, and should only be regarded as a guide in the absence of actual data, but it should none the less be useful. The examples in *Figs.* 3.2 and 3.3 show how the table might be used. Hopefully the increasing availability of empiric data for individual disorders should reduce the need for dependence on artificial models; wherever such data exist they should be used, even if they disagree with what is predicted from theory.

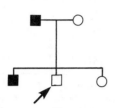

Fig. 3.2. The consultand (arrowed) has 1 sib and a parent with gastric cancer and wishes to know the risk of developing the disorder. No underlying Mendelian disorder or other causative factors have been found.

The disorder falls into the high frequency, but low heritability group, and the appropriate risk can be seen to be only 3·3 per cent. By contrast if the disorder were one of high heritability, the equivalent risk would be 18·5 per cent.

Fig. 3.3. An epileptic woman has 2 epileptic children and wishes to know the risk for her current pregnancy. Again, there is no specific cause to be found, and the effects of drugs are ignored in this example. Assigning appropriate categories is rather arbitrary here; heritability is probably high, but the frequency falls between the two categories; a risk of 20–25 per cent would be appropriate.

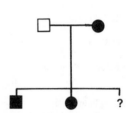

The Identification of Specific Genetic Factors in Common Diseases

The present situation in genetic counselling for most common disorders not following Mendelian inheritance is an unsatisfactory one; it is rarely possible to identify definite specific environmental or genetic factors, or to say whether a given case of the disease has resulted predominantly from an excess of genetic factors. The risks to relatives are generally low compared with those for Mendelian disorders, but not so low as to be comfortably ignored by families in which an affected individual has occurred. In the past few years, however, the situation has begun to change, and it is likely that we will soon be able to identify a variety of factors which will modify the 'empiric' risks based on overall population studies. It is perhaps easiest to explain this by using an example, that of ankylosing spondylitis (*see also* Chapter 11).

Until 1970, no specific genetic or environmental factors were known for ankylosing spondylitis; nevertheless family studies[4] had shown an empiric risk of around 4 per cent in sibs. The discovery of a strong association between the disease and the HLA antigen B27 made it clear that the HLA region was one of the main genetic determinants of the disease, possibly the most important one; 95 per cent of individuals with ankylosing spondylitis were found to possess HLA B27, compared with 7 per cent of normal individuals; conversely B27 individuals were 100–200 times more likely to have ankylosing spondylitis than those not possessing the antigen.

This information is in itself not enough to help in genetic counselling. What we need to know is: given that a patient with ankylosing spondylitis has B27, what are the risks for his sibs, children or other relatives developing the disease if they:

a. Have the B27 antigen.

b. Do not have the B27 antigen.

Table 3.4. HLA disease associations (based on Bodmer[5])

| | | Frequency (%) | | |
Disease	Antigen	Patients	Controls	Relative risk
Coeliac disease	Dw3	96	27	64·5
	B8	67	20	8·1
Active chronic hepatitis	DRw3	41	17	3·4
	B8	52	15	6·1
Myasthenia gravis	DRw3	32	17	2·3
	B8	39	17	3·1
Graves' disease	Dw3	53	18	5·1
	B8	44	18	3·6
Juvenile onset diabetes	DRw3	27	17	1·8
	B8	32	16	2·5
	DRw4	39	15	3·6
Rheumatoid arthritis	DRw4	56	15	7·2
Myasthenia gravis (Japanese)	DRw4	59	35	2·7
Juvenile onset diabetes (Japanese)	DRw4	65	35	3·4
Multiple sclerosis	DRw2	41	22	2·5
Ankylosing spondylitis	B27	90	8	103·5
Reiter's disease	B27	80	9	40·4
Haemochromatosis	A3	72	21	9·7
Psoriasis: caucasoids	Cw6	50	23	3·3
	B13	23	5	5·7
	B17	19	9	2·4
	B37	5	2	2·6
Psoriasis: Japanese	Cw6	53	7	15
	B13	18	1	22
	B37	35	2	26
	A1	30	2	21

The results of family studies confirm that the B27 first-degree relatives are indeed at considerably increased risk (9 per cent), whereas those without B27 are at low risk (under 1 per cent) – much lower than the figure that would have been given on the basis of family studies alone. The combined use of the different types of genetic information has resulted in an improved discrimination between those at high and those at low risks.

A number of important HLA associations are now known, and some are listed in Table 3.4. A clear review is given by Bodmer[5].

Unfortunately, information on how these associations affect the risks within the individual family is not yet available for most of these, though it should not be long before it is. Other associations (as with the ABO blood groups) are rarely strong enough to be of practical use in genetic counselling.

Genetic associations are often confused with genetic linkage, which implies a physical proximity of the genetic loci on the same chromosome. Some of the HLA associations listed in *Table* 3.4 may indeed result from actual linkage, especially where no immunological or other causative process exists that can explain the association of phenotypes. It is important to recognize that linkage of genetic loci, even when close, does not necessarily imply that an association will be found between a disease and a particular phenotype. The use of genetic linkage predictions in genetic counselling is more applicable to Mendelian than to multifactorial disorders and is discussed in Chapter 6.

References

1. Smith C. (1972) Computer programme to estimate recurrence risks for multi-factorial familial disease. *Br. Med. J.* **1**, 495–497.
2. Morton N. E., Yee S. and Elston R. C. (1970) Discontinuity and quasi-continuity: Alternative hypotheses of multifactorial inheritance. *Clin. Genet.* **1**, 81–94.
3. Smith C. (1971) Recurrence risks for multifactorial inheritance. *Am. J. Hum. Genet.* **23**, 578–588.
4. Emery A. E. H. and Lawrence J. S. (1967) Genetics of ankylosing spondylitis. *J. Med. Genet.* **4**, 239–244.
5. Bodmer W. F. (1980) The HLA system and disease. *J. R. Coll. Physicians Lond.* **14**, 43–50.

Further Reading

Carter C. O. (1976) Genetics of common single malformations. *Br. Med. Bull.* **32**, 21–26.
Carter C. O. (1977) Risk data. How good is empiric information? In: Lubs H. A. and De La Gruz F. (ed.), *Genetic Counselling.* New York, Raven Press.

CHAPTER FOUR

Chromosomal Abnormalities

Before describing the risks in specific groups of chromosomal disorders there are two facts that the clinician must bear in mind from the outset.

1. The great majority of chromosomal disorders have an extremely low risk of recurrence in a family.

2. The great majority of clearly hereditary disorders show no recognizable chromosomal abnormality.

It follows that while a very large number of chromosomal disorders has been described and while human cytogenetics is of fundamental importance in medical genetics, chromosomal disorders and chromosomal studies play a rather less important role in genetic counselling than is sometimes supposed. However, since chromosomal disorders are poorly treatable but eminently detectable by amniocentesis, it is essential that the small number of high-risk situations is clearly distinguished from the much larger number where the risk is low.

Chromosomal Terminology

The clinician whose knowledge of chromosomes is limited to the fact that 46 is the normal number and that males are XY is likely to be confused when he receives a report stating that his patient has:

$$45,XXt. (14q + 21-).$$

In fact interpreting reports or published papers is not too difficult if one remembers the following points:

1. The total chromosome number is stated first.
2. The sex chromosome constitution comes next,

    e.g. 46,XX   Normal female karyotype.

    47,XXY   Klinefelter syndrome.
3. An extra autosome is indicated by its number and a + ,

    e.g. 47,XY,21+   Male with trisomy 21.

    Loss of a whole autosome is correspondingly indicated by a −.
4. The short arm of a chromosome is indicated by the letter p (petit − due to the strong French influence in cytogenetics).

    The long arm is denoted by q.

    e.g. 46,XY,5p−   Deletion of short arm of chromosome 5 (as seen in Cri du Chat syndrome).

5. Translocations are denoted by t. with details in brackets,
   e.g. 45,XXt. (14q+21−) a female balanced 14/21 carrier − our
   original example, which is now seen to be quite logical!
6. The presence of more than one cell line (mosaicism) is indicated by
   a /,
   e.g. 45X/46XX   A mosaic for Turner's syndrome.

Further refinements allow one to deal with isochromosomes, ring
chromosomes, inversions and the identification of particular bands, but in
a complex situation a laboratory report will almost certainly describe the
abnormality in words as well. Wherever possible the clinician should visit
the laboratory and see the appearance himself. This will provide a more
meaningful idea of the problem and will allow a better assessment of risks
by discussion with his cytogeneticist colleagues. He will also find that they
are delighted at the chance to learn more about the clinical aspects, being
all too often cut off from direct contact with patients and their families.

A Normal Frequency of Chromosomal Abnormalities in the Population

Three sources of information are available:

   a. Studies of newborn populations.
   b. Studies of particular chromosomal disorders.
   c. Studies of abortions and stillbirths.

Table 4.1. Chromosome abnormalities in unselected Newborns (based on Jacobs et al.[1])

Abnormality	Frequency (per 1000)
All abnormalities	5·6
Autosomal trisomies	1·7
Balanced autosomal rearrangements	1·9
Other autosomal abnormalities	0·4
Sex chromosome abnormalities	
In phenotypic males	3·0
In phenotypic females	1·8

Studies of Unselected Newborn Populations

Table 4.1 summarizes the principal findings, based on the study of Jacobs
et al.[1]. It can be seen that 5·6/1000 or rather more than 1 in 200
infants had recognizable chromosomal abnormalities, of which around
2/1000 had autosomal abnormalities and a comparable number sex
chromosome abnormalities. Balanced autosomal rearrangements accounted
for a further 2/1000. Although the numbers were insufficient to give
accurate data on individual disorders, these figures are a useful reference
point with which to compare any increased risk. *Table* 4.2 gives data
collected on the major specific chromosome disorders while in *Tables* 4.3

and 4.4 data on spontaneous abortions are summarized. It can be seen that liveborn infants with chromosomal disorders represent only a small fraction of those conceived with such abnormalities. Indeed spontaneous abortion is the rule rather than the exception for most serious autosomal disorders, some of which (e.g. trisomy 16) are extremely common in abortuses, but rarely reach full-term. The incidence of chromosomal

Table 4.2. Population frequency of specific chromosomal disorders

	Per 1000 live births
Trisomy 21	1·5
Trisomy 18	0·12
Trisomy 13	0·07
XXY (Klinefelter syndrome)	2·0
XO (Turner syndrome)	0·4
XYY syndrome	1·5
XXX syndrome	0·65

Table 4.3. Chromosome abnormalities in spontaneous abortions and stillbirths (based on Carr and Gedeon[2])

	%
All spontaneous abortions	50
Up to 12 weeks	60
12–20 weeks	20
Stillbirths	5

Table 4.4. Major types of chromosome abnormality in spontaneous abortions (after Carr and Gedeon[2])

	%
Trisomies	52
XO	18
Triploidy	17
Translocations	2–4

abnormalities in abortions declines with increasing gestation, and studies of stillbirths have shown a frequency of around 5 per cent. Identification of a chromosomal abnormality in a stillbirth is of considerable practical importance, especially when multiple malformations are present, because it allows a possible rare Mendelian disorder to be ruled out.

Recurrence of Chromosomal Disorders in a Family

The chance of this is extremely low (not more than 1 per cent) in all the disorders listed in *Table* 4.2, provided that there is no parental chromosome abnormality and that no other risk factor (e.g. maternal age) exists. The most notable exception is for translocations (*see below*), but several particular situations require mention.

Trisomy 21

Most cases of Down's syndrome result from this, and the overall population incidence is around 1 in 650 live births. There is a well recognized (but often misinterpreted) relationship with maternal age shown in *Table* 4.5.

Table 4.5. Risk of Down's syndrome in relation to maternal age (live birth figures calculated for individual years)

Maternal age at delivery	Incidence (per 1000 births)	Risk
All ages	1·5	1 in 650
30	1·4	1 in 700
34	2·0	1 in 500
35	2·2	1 in 450
36	2·5	1 in 400
37	4·0	1 in 250
38	5·0	1 in 200
39	6·5	1 in 150
40	10·0	1 in 100
41	12·5	1 in 80
42	16·5	1 in 60
43	20	1 in 50
44	25	1 in 40

The risk figures are based on two large surveys, in Sweden[3] and Australia[4], as well as on a local study of births in South Glamorgan, the Cardiff Births Survey. (Data kindly provided by Dr I. D. Young and Dr E. M. Williams.)
The incidence figures given are approximate and are rounded off to be suitable for counselling.

Although a higher incidence has been suggested on the basis of amniocentesis data (*Table* 4.6) there is little doubt that the figures given here are valid for live births with Down's syndrome, and that they apply to most populations.

Several points are important to note:

1. The incidence in offspring of young women (25 and under) is very low (under 1 in 1000); it may rise again slightly in the youngest mothers.

2. The risk does not rise above that of the overall population risk until a maternal age of around 30.

3. The risk is around 1 in 200 (0·5 per cent) at age 38 years.

Table 4.6. Incidence of chromosomal
abnormalities found at amniocentesis
in relation to maternal age (based on
Ferguson-Smith[5])

| | Rate per 1000 births | |
	Downs	All abnormalities
35	4·5	7·5
36	4·9	9·8
37	7·7	13·4
38	9·1	14·6
39	13·2	18·6
40	12·0	23·3
41	23·4	30·6
42	33·3	61·0
43	17·8	40·6
44	55·9	76·9
45	33·5	50·3
46	81·0	135·1

4. The risk reaches 1 per cent at about 39 years of age and rises steeply
thereafter.

Recurrent Trisomy 21
The risk of another affected child being born to a couple who have had 1
trisomic Down's child is increased over the normal risk, but the increase
seems to be slight between a maternal age of 25–35 and greater at both
extremes. Confirmation of a low overall recurrence risk comes from
combined amniocentesis data[6] which showed a risk of 1 in 200 or 0·5
per cent for Down's syndrome and of 1 per cent for all chromosomal
abnormalities in pregnancies where the indication for amniocentesis was a
previous child with trisomy 21. Since live birth and amniocentesis data are
similar here, an appropriate risk for Down's syndrome recurring is 1 in 200
under age 35 and twice the normal age specific risk from 35 upwards. The
risk of all chromosome aberrations would be around double that for
Down's syndrome.

Risk for Offspring of Down's Patients
These would be expected to be high for both trisomic and translocation
patients, but data are scanty. A risk of around 1/3 for offspring of female
patients seems likely. There is no satisfactory information for mosaics.

Other Autosomal Trisomies (13, 18 and 22)
These are rare (as live births) in comparison with trisomy. Recurrence is
rare but data are few; maternal age is also a risk factor, but most of the
risk is for the commoner Down's syndrome and the risks given in *Table* 4.5
should be used. The only condition of high genetic risk is the small extra

chromosome fragment identified as part of 22, which may be associated with anal atresia and colobomas[7] and where transmission to offspring has been recorded.

Non-viable autosomal trisomies are extremely common in spontaneous abortions and it may be asked if amniocentesis is warranted if such an abnormality is detected. How far risks for a future liveborn child are increased by a previous chromosomally abnormal abortion is still uncertain; if the abnormality was a late abortion or stillbirth then it seems wise at present to use the same risk figures as for a livebirth.

Sex Chromosome Abnormalities

Recurrence in a family is exceptional for any of these. Even among the offspring of affected fertile individuals transmission is rare, for reasons not fully understood.

The XXY and XXX syndromes (but not XYY and XO) show a relation to maternal age. Predicting whether an individual with XYY or XXY karyotype found incidentally in a newborn (or at amniocentesis) will be phenotypically normal or not is extremely uncertain, but the mean intelligence of XXX females is significantly reduced.

The XO (Turner) syndrome is often accompanied by few clinical abnormalities other than hypogonadism in liveborn individuals, but is one of the commonest causes of spontaneous abortion.

Chromosomal Translocations

The great majority of cases of Down's syndrome have 47 chromosomes due to trisomy 21, but in about 5 per cent of cases the chromosome number is normal (46) and the extra chromosomal material is translocated onto another chromosome. Most commonly this is chromosome 14, less commonly chromosome 22. Very occasionally two 21 chromosomes are translocated onto each other.

The genetic risks in such a situation depend entirely on whether there is an abnormality in the parental chromosomes. If they are normal, the risk to further offspring is minimal[8] — the risks are probably similar to those following a trisomic child at a particular maternal age. If one parent has an abnormal karyotype the situation is entirely different.

The usual parental abnormality is a *balanced translocation,* in which the chromosome number is 45, but the total amount of chromosomal material is normal; one 21 will be absent, and an abnormal chromosome will be seen composed of the 21 and the chromosome onto which it has been translocated. Banding techniques will allow precise identification.

The possibilities for offspring of such a parent are shown in *Fig.* 4.1. In theory, one would expect all four categories of translocation Down's, normal, balanced translocation carrier and monosomy 21 to occur in equal proportions, but since the absence of one 21 (monosomy 21) is lethal and rarely results in an identified pregnancy, the risk of a child with

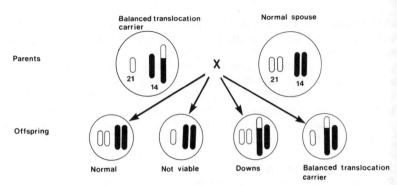

Fig. 4.1. Possibilities for offspring of a balanced 14/21 translocation carrier.

Table 4.7. Risks of abnormal liveborn offspring in families with translocation Down's syndrome

Type of translocation	Parent carrying balanced translocation	Risk to offspring (%)
14/21	Mother	10
	Father	2·5
	Neither parent	<1
21/22	One parent	Data scanty, risks probably as for 14/21 translocation
	Neither parent	Very low, (probably <1)
21/21	One parent (either sex)	100
	Neither parent	Very low, (probably <1)

translocation Down's syndrome should be 1/3. In fact it is considerably less, particularly when the father is carrying the balanced translocation. *Table* 4.7 summarizes the risks.

Two cautions should be given regarding these risks: first, the risk of an abnormality detected at amniocentesis is higher than in *Table* 4.7 probably around 1 in 8 for pregnancies of a woman who is a balanced 14/21 translocation carrier. Secondly, data have been obtained principally from women who have already had an abnormal child — where the balanced chromosomal abnormality is detected incidentally the risk may well be less.

Data for the rarer 21/22 translocation are much less extensive than for 14/21, but risks are probably equivalent. However, in the case of the rare (and genetically lethal) 21/21 translocation *all* pregnancies will be abnormal since the only alternatives are the unbalanced translocation Down's and the lethal monosomy (*Fig.* 4.2).

Once a case of translocation Down's syndrome has been identified it is essential to test all close relatives to identify unsuspected balanced translocation carriers (of both sexes), who can then be offered amniocentesis in any future pregnancy. It is rare now for a case of Down's syndrome *not* to be karyotyped, but clearly this is especially important in the infants of

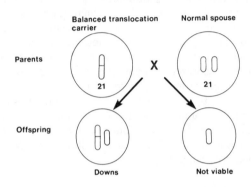

Fig. 4.2. Possibilities for offspring of a balanced 21/21 translocation carrier. All viable offspring of such an individual will have Down's syndrome.

younger mothers, in whom trisomy is less frequent (though it is commoner than translocation at all ages). A register of both translocations and trisomies will often save unnecessary amniocentesis in relatives at a later date.

Other Translocations

Not all translocations are found during the investigation of Down's syndrome. Some may be responsible for other multiple malformation syndromes, or parental abnormalities may be discovered as a result of chromosomal studies for recurrent abortion or infertility (*see* Chapter 19). The individual situation will need careful study, but the following general points can be made.

1. The recurrence risk of an abnormality is only high if one of the parents is a balanced carrier for the translocation.

2. If the rearrangement in the propositus appears balanced, it should be questioned whether it is related to the condition in question. Study of the family may help by showing healthy members with the chromosome 'abnormality'.

3. Balanced D–D group translocations are relatively common and are not usually associated with unbalanced chromosome defects in the offspring. By contrast translocations involving chromosome 9 appear to have a high risk of an unbalanced defect (possibly as high as 30 per cent).

Otherwise recurrence risks are approximately those given in *Table* 4.7 for 14/21 translocation Down's syndrome.

Inversions

Rearrangement of genetic material within a chromosome is relatively common, usually harmless to the individual concerned, and increasingly recognized by chromosome banding techniques. When the rearrangement is confined to one arm of a chromosome there is not likely to be any risk of abnormality in the offspring; however, if the centromere is involved this will cause problems in pairing of chromosomes at meiosis and gametes with an unbalanced chromosome complement may be formed. This situation may be discovered in a parent after a child with an unbalanced chromosome abnormality has been born, or it may be an incidental finding. Figures are very scanty as to the risks of abnormality; where an abnormal child has been born amniocentesis is wise in future pregnancies, but where it is an incidental discovery it is much less certain whether there is a significant increase in risk. The situation should be discussed carefully with the cytogenetics laboratory.

Mosaicism

In mosaics more than one cell line is present. This may cause difficulty in diagnosis because the abnormal line may be missed on a single (or even repeated) blood study. Difficulty in counselling results from the fact that such patients more frequently reproduce (because of the milder clinical picture) than do patients with full chromosome anomalies, and because of uncertainty as to whether the germ cell-line is involved. There are no accurate risk figures for offspring, but amniocentesis is indicated.

Other Chromosome Abnormalities

For details of these the reader should consult the books on cytogenetics listed at the end of this chapter. All the following disorders are of low recurrence risk from the viewpoint of counselling, but are mentioned since genetic advice may well be requested when they have occurred in a family.

Deletions involve loss of a part of a chromosome. Phenotypic features are less severe than when an entire chromosome is lost, so they are seen not infrequently as live births. Banding techniques have identified a number of small deletions not recognizable with previous techniques.

Ring chromosomes are essentially deletions in which the two ends of the abnormal chromosomes have joined together.

Isochromosomes. These are most commonly seen for the X chromosome and result from faulty separation of chromatids so that a symmetrical chromosome consisting of either two long arms or two short arms is formed.

References

1. Jacobs P. A., Melville M., Ratcliffe S. et al. (1974) A cytogenetic survey of 11,680 newborn infants. *Ann. Hum. Genet.* **37**, 359–376.
2. Carr D. H. and Gedeon M. (1977) Population cytogenetics of human abortuses. In: Hook E. B. and Porter I. H. (ed.), *Population Cytogenetics. Studies in Human.* New York, Academic Press.
3. Hook E. B. and Lindsjo A. (1978) Down syndrome in live births by single year maternal age interval in a Swedish study. *Am. J. Hum. Genet.* **30**, 19–27.
4. Sutherland G. R., Clisby S. R., Bloor G. et al. (1979) Down's syndrome in South Australia. *Med. J. Aust.* **2**, 58–61.
5. Ferguson-Smith M. A. (1979) Maternal age specific incidence of chromosome aberrations at amniocentesis. In: Murken J. D., Stengel-Rutkowski S. and Schwinger E. (ed), *Prenatal Diagnosis,* Stuttgart, Enke, pp. 1–14.
6. Mikkelsen M. (1979) Previous child with Down syndrome and other chromosome aberration. In: Murken J. D., Stengel-Rutkowski S. and Schwinger E. (ed.), *Prenatal Diagnosis,* Stuttgart, Enke, pp. 22–29.
7. Gerald P. S., Davis C., Say B. et al. (1972) Syndromal associations of imperforate anus: the Cat Eye syndrome. *Birth Defects.* **8**, No. 2, pp. 79–84.
8. Gardner R. J. M. and Veale A. M. O. (1974) De novo translocation Down's syndrome: risk of recurrence of Down's syndrome. *Clin. Genet.* **6**, 160–164.

Further Reading

de Grouchy J. and Turleau C. (1977) *Clinical Atlas of Human Chromosomes.* New York, John Wiley.
Hamerton J. L. (1971) *Human Cytogenetics. Vol. 2 Clinical Cytogenetics.* New York, Academic Press.
Smith G. F. and Berg J. M. (1976) *Down's Anomaly.* London, Churchill Livingstone.
Valentine G. H. (1975) *The Chromosome Disorders. An Introduction for Clinicians.* Philadelphia, Lippincott. 3rd ed.
Yunis J. J. (ed.) (1979) *New Chromosomal Syndromes.* New York, Academic Press.

CHAPTER FIVE

Carrier Detection in Genetic Disorders

One of the major tasks in genetic counselling is to identify those individuals who, while apparently healthy themselves, have a high risk of transmitting a genetic disorder. Recognition of a particular mode of inheritance will often allow the risk to be estimated and in some cases excluded, but where the risk is high it is rarely possible to tell with certainty whether a particular family member does or does not possess the abnormal gene. For this reason, tests which will identify the correct genotype of a person are of great importance and in many instances form an integral part of the overall process of genetic counselling. This chapter explores the range and limitations of tests of carrier detection and attempts to show how the information can be used in conjunction with other genetic data in making as accurate prediction as possible.

What is a Carrier?

The term 'carrier' is widely used in medicine, and is often applied to those harbouring an infective agent, quite apart from its use in Medical Genetics. The term may be used by different people with quite different connotations, and a precise definition is important if confusion is not to arise. A working definition of the carrier state in inherited disease is:

'A carrier is an individual who possesses in heterozygous state the gene determining an inherited disorder, and who is essentially healthy at the time of study.'

From this definition several important points follow:

1. A carrier is a heterozygote; thus the term can only be applied satisfactorily to Mendelian disorders determined by a single locus.

It is logical to talk about a carrier for cystic fibrosis, but not of a carrier for spina bifida, where the genetic determination is poorly understood and non-Mendelian. The definition can, however, be stretched to individuals with a balanced chromosomal abnormality, such as a translocation, where the inheritance is essentially Mendelian (*see* Chapter 4).

2. Although a carrier is heterozygous this does not necessarily imply that the affected individual must be homozygous. This will only be the case in autosomal recessive disorders; in autosomal dominant disorders essentially all individuals, whether affected or carriers, will be heterozygous.

3. Although the risk of a carrier transmitting the abnormal gene is high

(normally 50 per cent), it does not always follow that there is a high risk of having an affected child. The risk may in fact be extremely low and will depend on the mode of inheritance (*Table* 5.1).

4. The fact that a carrier is 'essentially healthy' at the time of study does not mean that minor clinical features may not be distinguishable, nor does it mean that the individual will necessarily remain healthy. Those carrying the gene for Huntington's chorea provide an obvious example of the latter point.

It is clear from these considerations that carrier detection has to be approached in the light of the natural history of the particular genetic disorder and its mode of inheritance.

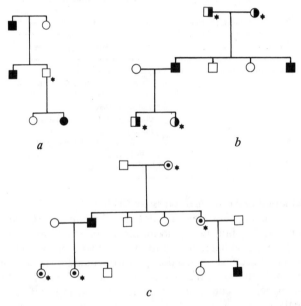

Fig. 5.1. Obligatory carriers in Mendelian inheritance. Obligatory carriers for the three major modes of inheritance are asterisked. By convention carriers for autosomal recessive disorders are half shaded, those for X-linked disorders dotted. *a*, Autosomal dominant inheritance. Any individual having both an affected parent and affected offspring must be a carrier. *b*, Autosomal recessive inheritance. Both parents and all offspring of an affected individual are obligatory carriers. *c*, X-linked recessive inheritance. Obligatory carriers include all daughters of an affected male and all women who have an affected son and at least one other affected male relative.

Obligatory and Possible Carriers

When the testing of carriers is being considered, it is often not recognized that in addition to individuals at a higher or lower risk of being a carrier, there are those who on genetic grounds *must* be a carrier (*Fig.* 5.1). Recognition of these 'obligatory' carriers is important for several reasons;

it may save complex and unnecessary testing procedures, it allows much more definite genetic counselling to be given, and also provides a reference population against which any new or improved carrier test can be evaluated. Obligatory carriers for autosomal recessive disorders include all children and parents of an affected individual (mutation as an alternative is too rare to be a practical problem); in X-linked recessive inheritance all daughters of an affected male will be obligatory carriers, while in autosomal dominant inheritance an obligatory carrier is a person who has both a parent and offspring affected but who shows (or showed when alive) no abnormalities himself. This situation is commonly seen in Huntington's chorea when an individual has died young of an unrelated cause, but is later shown to have transmitted the disorder.

Table 5.1. Genetic risks for carriers of Mendelian disorders

Inheritance	Risk to offspring of carrier
Autosomal recessive	Very low unless a. disorder is extremely common or b. same disorder or consanguinity in spouse's family;
Autosomal dominant	50% (risk of overt disease will vary with disorder)
X-linked recessive	50% of male offspring affected

Carrier Detection in Autosomal Recessive Disease

Autosomal recessive disorders provide by far the largest number of carriers numerically, but are by no means the most important in genetic counselling. We are all likely to be carriers for at least one serious recessive disorder and several lethal ones, quite apart from numerous polymorphisms where heterozygosity is normal and almost certainly beneficial. From the standpoint of genetic counselling there are three main situations that are encountered.

1. An individual is or is likely to be a carrier for a rare autosomal recessive disorder.

2. An individual is or is likely to be a carrier for a common autosomal recessive disorder.

3. The situation is complicated by consanguinity or by marriage to an individual whose family may be affected by the same disorder.

The importance or lack of importance of the carrier state in these three situations is directly related to the principles of autosomal recessive inheritance which have been discussed in Chapter 2.

Rare autosomal recessive disorders are those about which advice is most commonly sought, and family members may be greatly worried and alarmed by having been told they may be carriers in this situation. Such worry (usually induced by doctors in the first place) is entirely unnecessary, but is often extremely difficult to allay. Some individuals may believe that being a carrier means one has the disease in a mild form, or is in some way not entirely healthy. Others believe that even though healthy themselves, their children will inevitably be affected.

Neither situation is of course, the case. Heterozygotes for autosomal recessive disorders are almost always entirely healthy and will remain so, even when minor distinguishing features can be found. Likewise even though the chance of the sibs of affected individuals, who are those most commonly seeking advice, being carriers is two-thirds, the risk of such

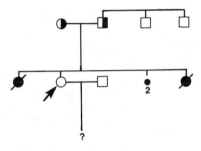

Fig. 5.2. Carrier detection in a rare autosomal recessive disorder – cystinosis. The sister of the two children who had died from cystinosis sought genetic advice during her first pregnancy to know what was the risk of being a carrier herself and of having affected offspring. Although the chance of her being a carrier is high (2/3), the risk of an affected child is minimal since her husband would also have to be a carrier for this rare gene. They were advised that neither carrier detection (which is unreliable) nor prenatal diagnosis (which carries a significant risk) were justified in this situation. A healthy boy was subsequently born.

carriers having affected children is exceptionally low, as shown in *Table* 2.2, p. 33, and for all rare autosomal recessive disorders a confident reassurance can be given. Some family members may request carrier testing for themselves and their spouses, if this is feasible, 'just to be sure'. In general the author discourages this, since for most rare inborn errors of metabolism where testing is possible, it is likely that the margin of error of the test greatly exceeds the risk of offspring being affected. Prenatal diagnosis is similarly rarely justified.

An example of this type of situation may be given: A woman whose two brothers had died from the rare autosomal recessive disorder cystinosis was seen for genetic counselling in her first pregnancy. The question of prenatal diagnosis was raised, but it was pointed out that though she had a two-thirds chance of being a carrier, the maximum risk of an affected child was 1 in 500, and that the risk of an erroneous result of prenatal diagnosis was likely to be considerably greater than this (*Fig.* 5.2).

Common autosomal recessive disorders provide a much more important indication for carrier detection, though it can again be seen from *Table* 2.2, p. 33 that the disorders have to be extremely common to present a significant risk to individual couples. Even for a disorder as relatively common as phenylketonuria (1 in 10 000 births) the risk for offspring of a healthy sib is only 1 in 300. Very few of the classic enzyme deficiencies for which carrier testing is available are as common as this, except for special concentrations such as Tay—Sachs disease in Ashkenazi Jewish populations. The haemoglobinopathies and thalassaemias provide the most important group on a worldwide basis, and carrier detection is fortunately feasible in most of these. *Table* 5.2 lists some of the major disorders in this

Table 5.2. Carrier detection in some common autosomal recessive disorders

Sickle-cell disease	Sickle test, Hb electrophoresis
Thalassaemias	Hb electrophoresis, blood film
Tay—Sachs disease (Ashkenazi Jews)	Hexosaminidase A assay (serum and WBC)
Cystic fibrosis	Not feasible at present
Phenylketonuria	Phenylalanine load, phenyl-alanine: tyrosine ratio

group; it should be noted that in cystic fibrosis (where more tests of carrier detection have probably been described than in all the others put together) none is currently (1980) reliable enough for clinical use.

When carrier testing for one of the commoner autosomal recessive disorders is being undertaken it is logical to test both the family member at risk and the spouse (or prospective spouse) at the same time, since if only one proves to be a carrier the couple can confidently be reassured. Where an individual affected with an autosomal recessive disorder is concerned, only the spouse need, of course, be tested.

Consanguinity may occasionally produce the need for carrier testing in a rare disorder where the risks would otherwise be negligible; even more rarely the same disorder may be present in the families of two unrelated partners. The heterozygote can be distinguished in the case of numerous rare inborn errors of metabolism, but it should be noted that there is often considerable overlap between the normal and heterozygote ranges, so that a clear indication of the likely margin of error should be obtained from the laboratory involved.

To conclude, it can be seen that for autosomal recessive disorders, the time and energy of the person involved in genetic counselling should normally be employed in a clear explanation of the (usually very low) risks and the *lack of importance* of being a carrier, rather than in attempting difficult, expensive and generally unnecessary tests of carrier detection. As with any test carrying a significant margin of error, it should only be employed in a situation where the prior risk is sufficiently high to warrant it.

Autosomal Dominant Inheritance

For practical purposes all individuals with a dominantly inherited disease are heterozygotes, so the carrier state can only exist where the disorder is mild, variable, or late in onset. One cannot be a carrier for achondroplasia — one either has it or does not. Thus, the number of dominantly inherited disorders where carrier detection is applicable is much less than for those following autosomal recessive inheritance, but the importance in terms of risks to offspring is much greater.

Table 5.3. Carrier detection in autosomal dominant disorders

Familial hypercholesterolaemia	Serum lipoprotein electrophoresis and cholesterol
Hereditary spherocytosis	Red cell osmotic fragility
Acute intermittent porphyria	Red cell uroporphyrinogen synthetase assay
Variegate porphyria	Faecal porphyrin excretion
Myotonic dystrophy	Electromyography, slit-lamp examination
Huntington's chorea	Not feasible at present
Osteogenesis imperfecta	Radiology, audiometry
Polycystic kidney disease (adult)	Ultrasound, pyelography

Table 5.3 lists some of the major autosomal dominant disorders where carrier detection is feasible, and it can be seen that there are three principal categories. The first are disorders which frequently remain asymptomatic and which under normal circumstances might hardly be considered diseases. The acute porphyrias and malignant hyperpyrexia, all drug-aggravated disorders, are examples. The second group consists of those difficult disorders which show variable penetrance and expression, and which are especially important in genetic counselling because of this variability. Tuberous sclerosis, osteogenesis imperfecta (*Fig.* 5.3) and myotonic dystrophy all fall into this class. The final group consists of diseases which sooner or later follow regular dominant inheritance, but where the true state of affairs may not be clear at the time when individuals at risk wish to have children. Huntington's chorea (Chapter 10) is far and away the most important and most difficult disorder in this group, but some of the other progressive neurological degenerations are comparable. Here tests of carrier detection are essentially tests of presymptomatic diagnosis.

In contrast to autosomal recessive disorders, the risk of the offspring of a carrier for an autosomal dominant condition having overt disease at some stage of their life is high. Although in a few cases (e.g. the myopathy

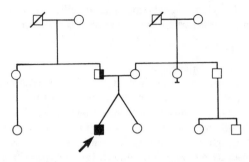

Fig. 5.3. Carrier detection in a variable autosomal dominant disorder – osteogenesis imperfecta. The propositus, a dizygotic twin, sustained a fractured femur during delivery and developed seven further major fractures over the subsequent two years; the typical clinical features of moderately severe osteogenesis imperfecta were present. Neither parent showed any skeletal abnormalities, but the father had progressive sensorineural deafness of otosclerotic type similar to that encountered in osteogenesis imperfecta. No other family members were affected. Although the possibility could not be ruled out that the child represented a new mutation and that the father's deafness was coincidental, it was considered more likely that he was carrying the gene for osteogenesis imperfecta, with a consequent 50 per cent risk for subsequent children. The couple subsequently decided to have no further children.

underlying malignant hyperpyrexia) the disorder remains constantly subclinical in successive generations, it is common to find severely affected offspring born to carrier parents. This in part reflects the natural variability of these disorders, but also results from the fact that the carrier parents form the mildest extreme of a range of variability, so that in 'reverting to the mean' the children are more likely to be clinically affected. In some instances, as with myotonic dystrophy and possibly neurofibromatosis, there may be maternal effects producing severe disease in the offspring of an asymptomatic mother.

Autosomal dominant disorders of late onset also produce a special difficulty in carrier detection since, in contrast to those with a static course, and to recessively inherited disease, the carrier is not just at risk of transmitting the disease but of developing it. Thus to identify an individual as a carrier for Huntington's chorea (not definitely feasible at present) would inevitably mark out that person as being destined to develop the disease at some time in the future. It is debatable whether this information would be acceptable to many individuals, and whether they would still wish for a test of carrier status carrying this knowledge with it, even though it would undoubtedly help those who proved to be normal and who cannot at present be distinguished from those carrying the gene.

X-linked Disorders
A relatively small number of X-linked recessive disorders provide the most important of all applications of carrier detection. The reason for this is

simple; the carriers are generally healthy and will so be likely to reproduce, but in contrast to autosomal recessive inheritance, they will be at risk of having affected male offspring regardless of whom they marry. In such a situation the availability of carrier detection for women at high risk is a major contribution, and forms such an integral part of genetic counselling that it is often of little purpose fully discussing the risks until information from testing is available.

Table 5.4. Carrier detection in Duchenne muscular dystrophy and haemophilia

	Duchenne muscular dystrophy	*Haemophilia A*
Clinical abnormalities (when present)	Minor weakness, often asymmetrical	Slight to moderate bleeding tendency
Principal test	Serum creatine kinase	Serum Factor VIII assays (immunological and functional)
Other tests	Muscle biopsy, ? red cell and lymphocyte defects	
Proportion of definite carriers showing results outside the normal range	Two-thirds	Around 80%

Haemophilia (principally haemophilia A) and X-linked muscular dystrophy (principally Duchenne dystrophy) are overwhelmingly the most important disorders that have to be considered in this group, and the approaches to carrier detection and the problems of interpretation are remarkably similar in each. For this reason, although details are given with the individual disorders, they will be used here as examples of carrier detection in X-linked recessive disease.

Table 5.4 summarizes some of the features. In both disorders a few carriers may be detectable clinically, probably as the result of X-chromosome inactivation having randomly resulted in a higher than expected proportion of those X-chromosomes bearing the abnormal gene functioning in the particular tissue of importance. Unfortunately, this process will also result in the opposite − namely carriers in whom principally the normal X chromosomes are functioning, and who will thus be difficult or even impossible to detect even by the most sensitive tests. This variability of X-linked carriers is characteristic and must always be borne in mind.

In some disorders, the problem of X-chromosome inactivation can be overcome, or even turned to advantage, by cloning cultured cells to separate out two populations, one of which will behave normally, the other abnormally. This is feasible in the Hunter syndrome, but is a complex procedure. A simpler, but less reliable approach is to use hair bulbs, which are usually derived from a single clone of cells having the same X chromosome active; the demonstration of two populations has been used to detect the carrier state in the Lesch–Nyhan and Hunter syndromes. Neither approach is currently feasible for haemophilia or Duchenne dystrophy.

The test generally used for Duchenne dystrophy, the elevation of serum creatine kinase, is considerably further removed from the basic molecular defect than the assays for Factor VIII in haemophilia, with consequently less precision in detecting carriers. In both disorders, however, there is a considerable overlap between normal and carrier ranges which makes it impossible to classify most individuals as 'normal' or 'abnormal'. Instead a series of likelihood ratios must be used which will give odds for or against the carrier state for any particular result of carrier test. By using these odds one can arrive at a much more precise separation of carriers and non-carriers than would otherwise be possible, especially if the results are integrated with other genetic information as described in Chapter 2. At the risk of repetition it must be stressed that the result of such a carrier test is *not* the same as the risk of being a carrier; its interpretation will vary depending on the genetic odds, and its use without these odds may result in serious error.

The isolated case of an X-linked disorder presents major problems in carrier detection. As discussed in Chapter 2, there is considerable uncertainty as to the proportion of such cases likely to represent new mutations, and correspondingly the proportion of mothers who are carriers. It is likely that this may vary from one disorder to another, even when reproduction of affected males does not occur. The prior risk of such a mother being a carrier will be somewhere between two-thirds and 1, and the interpretation of carrier testing will clearly be influenced by this figure.

All daughters of a man with an X-linked recessive disease *must* be carriers, and so tests of carrier detection are irrelevant for such people. Despite this, they are often referred for 'genetic counselling and carrier detection' under the misapprehension that a normal result will somehow make a definite carrier less definite! False reassurance is a real danger in such a situation.

Table 5.5 shows some of the X-linked recessive disorders where carrier detection is helpful. The range of approaches is wide and may be morphological, functional or biochemical. Taken as a group, X-linked disorders are probably the most satisfactory in terms of our ability to detect the carrier state and its applicability in preventing the disease within families.

Methods of Carrier Detection
The techniques available for detecting the carrier state vary greatly according to the nature of the particular disease and our understanding of its metabolic basis. It is impossible to give all the details here, and available approaches are mentioned as far as possible with individual disorders, but

Table 5.5. Carrier detection in X-linked disorders

Disorder	Abnormality in carrier
Duchenne muscular dystrophy [1] [2] [3]	Serum creatine kinase (*see* Chapter 9)
Becker muscular dystrophy [4]	Serum creatine kinase (less effective than in Duchenne)
Haemophilia A [5]	Factor VIII assays (*see* Chapter 21)
Haemophilia B [5]	Factor IX assay
Glucose-6-phosphate dehydrogenase deficiency	Quantitative enzyme assay and electrophoresis
Hunter's syndrome (MPS II) [6]	Enzyme assay or sulphate uptake on hair bulbs or cloned cells
Hypogammaglobulinaemia (Bruton type)	Reduced IgG
Fabry's disease [7]	Skin lesions; alphagalactosidase assay
Lesch–Nyhan syndrome [8]	HGPRT assay on hair bulbs
Vitamin D resistant rickets	Serum phosphate (may be clinical features)
X-linked mental retardation [9]	? visible fragile site on X chromosome
Lowe's syndrome [10]	Amino aciduria, lens opacities
X-linked congenital cataract	Lens opacities
Ocular albinism	Patchy fundal depigmentation
X-linked retinitis pigmentosa [11]	Pigmentary changes; abnormal electroretinogram
Choroideraemia	Pigmentary retinal changes
Retinoschisis	Cystic retinal changes
X-linked ichthyosis	Corneal opacities, reduced steroid sulphatase
Anhidrotic ectodermal dysplasia [12]	Reduced sweat pores, dental defects
Amelogenesis imperfecta	Patchy enamel hypoplasia

it is worth considering the broad forms of approach and some of the limitations which exist. *Table* 5.6 summarizes these.

1. Measurement of the primary enzyme or other defect. This is much the most satisfactory approach where available, and is feasible for numerous inborn errors of metabolism, mostly following autosomal recessive inheritance, as well as for non-enzymic defects such as haemophilia and various haemoglobinopathies. Even in this group, however, the range of results in heterozygotes may show considerable overlap with the normal range, and less commonly with that of the abnormal homozygotes. The appropriate tissue to use will also vary. Serum may be adequate but more often red or white blood cells or cultured fibroblasts are required, and the techniques may be difficult and specialised. X-linked disorders are particularly variable, as already discussed.

2. Secondary biochemical changes. The value of these will in general be related to how close the abnormality is to the primary defect. Important examples are the use of creatine kinase in Duchenne muscular dystrophy, elevation of fetal haemoglobin in β-thalassaemia, and abnormalities of faecal porphyrin excretion in the acute porphyrias. As our knowledge

Table 5.6. Approaches to carrier detection

	Example
1. Biochemical, primary defect known	
a. Enzyme deficiency	Hexosaminidase A (Tay–Sachs disease)
b. Non-enzymic protein defect	Factor VIII assays (haemophilia A)
2. Biochemical, primary defect	
a. Unknown	Serum creatine kinase (Duchenne muscular dystrophy)
b. Inaccessible	Phenylalanine load (phenylketonuria)
3. Physiological	
a. Electroretinography	X-linked retinitis pigmentosa
b. Electromyography	Muscular dystrophies (myotonic and Duchenne)
4. Microscopy	
a. Biopsy	Duchenne dystrophy
b. Chromosomal studies	Balanced translocation carriers
c. Ocular slit-lamp	X-linked ichthyosis, myotonic dystrophy
5. Radiology	Tuberous sclerosis (cerebral calcification)
6. Clinical	Skin (Fabry's disease)
	Eye (Choroideraemia)
	Muscle (Duchenne dystrophy)

increases, such tests will tend to be superseded or used as preliminary screening tests. Even when a disorder is thoroughly understood in enzymatic terms, a secondary test may be the most useful; thus in phenylketonuria the enzyme is confined to the liver, and carrier detection is usually achieved by studying the blood phenylalanine-tyrosine ratio under standardized conditions or by performing a phenylalanine loading test.

3. Physiological tests. These are of particular use in those autosomal dominant conditions where we have little biochemical understanding. Major examples include the use of electroretinography in detecting the carriers of X-linked retinitis pigmentosa and electromyography in myotonic dystrophy.

4. Microscopic techniques. These may rely on biopsy, as in Duchenne muscular dystrophy, blood film examination, as with sickle-cell anaemia or thalassaemias, or on biomicroscopy, as in slit-lamp examination for the lens opacities of myotonic dystrophy or the corneal opacities of X-linked ichthyosis.

5. Radiology. This may show minor skeletal abnormalities in such disorders as osteogenesis imperfecta, while internal defects may be visible, e.g. cerebral calcification and abnormal CT scan in tuberous sclerosis or pyelographic abnormalities in polycystic kidney disease.

6. Clinical observation. Many carriers may show some clinical evidence that shows their genotype and although the absence of such features rarely excludes an individual being a carrier, their presence provides strong positive evidence. Ophthalmic disorders (e.g. choroideraemia and retinitis

pigmentosa) are particularly susceptible to carrier detection in this way, as are skin disorders. Female carriers for an X-linked recessive disorder may show a 'patchy' appearance as already noted; again this is particularly evident in skin and eye disorders where the tissue concerned is open to inspection.

References

1. Emery A. E. H. (1969) Genetic counselling in X-linked muscular dystrophy. *J. Neurol. Sci.* **8**, 579–587.
2. Dennis N. R., Evans K., Clayton B. et al. (1976) Use of creatine kinase for detecting severe X-linked muscular dystrophy carriers. *Br. Med. J.* **2**, 577–579.
3. Sibert J. R., Harper P. S., Thompson R. J. et al. (1979) Carrier detection in Duchenne muscular dystrophy. Evidence from a study of obligatory carriers and mothers of isolated cases. *Arch. Dis. Child.* **54**, 534–537.
4. Skinner R., Emery A. E. H., Anderson A. J. B. et al. (1975) The detection of carriers of benign (Becker-type) X-linked muscular dystrophy. *J. Med. Genet.* **12**, 131–134.
5. Graham J. B. (1979) Genotype assignment (carrier detection) in the haemophilias. *Clin. Haematol.* **8**, 115–145.
6. Nwokoro N. and Neufeld E. (1979) Detection of Hunter heterozygotes by enzymatic analysis of hair roots. *Am. J. Hum. Genet.* **31**, 42–49.
7. Beaudet A. L. and Caskey C. T. (1978) Detection of Fabry's disease heterozygotes by hair root analysis. *Clin. Genet.* **13**, 251–258.
8. McKeran R. O., Andrews T. M., Howell A. et al. (1975) The diagnosis of the carrier state for the Lesch–Nyhan syndrome. *Q. J. Med.* **44**, 189–205.
9. Sutherland G. R. (1977) Fragile sites on human chromosomes: demonstration of their dependence on the type of tissue culture medium. *Science* **197**, 265–266.
10. Johnston S. S. and Nevin N. C. (1976) Ocular manifestations in patients and female relatives of families with the oculocerebrorenal syndrome of Lowe. In: Bergsma D., Bron A. J. and Cotlier E. (ed.), *The Eye and Inborn Errors of Metabolism*, New York, Alan Liss, pp. 569–577.
11. Warburg M. and Simonsen S. E. (1968) Sex-linked recessive retinitis pigmentosa. A preliminary study of the carriers. *Acta Ophthalmol.* **46**, 494–499.
12. Kerr C. B., Wells R. S. and Cooper K. E. (1966) Gene effect in carriers of anhidrotic ectodermal dysplasia. *J. Med. Genet.* **3**, 169–176.

CHAPTER SIX

Prenatal Diagnosis

The development of techniques for diagnosing certain genetic disorders in utero has proved to be a major advance in medical genetics, and has so altered the outlook for families at risk of having affected children that it has become an integral part of genetic counselling. Prenatal diagnostic procedures have frequently been developed by or in close association with those actively involved in genetic counselling, and perhaps as a result of this have in general been used appropriately and responsibly. The increasingly widespread use and diversified nature of the techniques is tending more recently to result in prenatal diagnostic procedures being applied as a substitute for genetic counselling, rather than as a powerful tool in supporting it. The author believes strongly that this is an unfortunate and potentially harmful trend, and that prenatal diagnosis, like other clinical and laboratory techniques, must be seen in the context of the entire situation — the risk of a pregnancy being genetically affected, the other measures such as carrier detection which may define that risk more precisely, the potential for treatment of the disorder in question and, most important, the attitude and wishes of the couple concerned.

Such an approach means that wherever possible prenatal diagnosis must be considered, discussed and planned *before* a pregnancy occurs. To leave this process until during pregnancy is highly undesirable (though sometimes inevitable) since not only may procedures have to be hurried, but most pregnant women (and their husbands) are not in a state where an objective assessment of the factors for or against prenatal diagnosis can be undertaken. It is likely that much of the emotional trauma sometimes associated with prenatal diagnosis results from absence of careful prior planning.

The Criteria and Indications for Prenatal Diagnosis
When prenatal diagnosis is being considered in genetic counselling, three basic factors must be examined:

1. Is the disorder sufficiently severe for this approach to be warranted?
2. Is an accurate prenatal diagnostic test feasible?
3. Are the genetic risks sufficient for prenatal diagnosis to be indicated in the particular situation under consideration?

Since most prenatal diagnostic procedures involve a large amount of worry (and a small amount of discomfort) to the mother, and a significant morbidity and mortality to the fetus (with 100 per cent mortality if the test proves abnormal), it should be obvious that prenatal diagnosis should not be considered unless a number of general criteria are fulfilled. These are summarized in *Table* 6.1 and are self-evident, but as in most clinical situations cases of real doubt may occur.

Table 6.1. Criteria for prenatal diagnosis

Disorder sufficiently severe to warrant termination of pregnancy
Treatment absent or unsatisfactory
Termination of pregnancy acceptable to the couple concerned
Accurate prenatal diagnostic test available
Genetic risk to pregnancy sufficiently high

Severity is beyond doubt in most of the disorders for which prenatal diagnosis is employed, including Down's syndrome and other autosomal trisomies, open neural tube defects and the rare neurodegenerative metabolic disorders. Other conditions may be more questionable, especially those where physical abnormalities (e.g. limb defects) may be accompanied by normal intellect and life expectancy. Such categories may be expected to increase and to present difficult decisions.

Treatment may be clear-cut and satisfactory in some disorders which might otherwise be considered for prenatal diagnosis. Thus in phenylketonuria (not currently detectable prenatally) most children now have near-normal health and intelligence; by contrast in galactosaemia occasional infants have liver damage present at birth. Whether prenatal diagnosis is undertaken here will probably depend on the attitudes and previous experience of the parents. In congenital adrenal hyperplasia (Chapter 19) a further factor results from the fact that the outlook with treatment for a second child is much better than for the first, in which delayed diagnosis commonly results in death or serious morbidity.

Acceptability of termination of pregnancy to a couple is essential to determine before any prenatal procedures are contemplated. In some cases it is unacceptable on religious grounds or because of the prevailing attitude of the community; in others, it is a more personal ethical view. Acceptability may be a relative phenomenon. Thus many couples find fetal sexing with termination of a male pregnancy which may be normal unacceptable, whereas these same individuals would accept termination of a *definitely* affected male pregnancy. It is essential to know the attitude of a couple before pregnancy occurs since this may well determine whether they decide for or against having further children.

The *feasibility* of prenatal diagnosis in a particular disorder is discussed in detail in later parts of this chapter, but it cannot be too strongly stressed that the clinician giving genetic counselling must obtain accurate information on this point *before* suggesting the possibility to a couple and must satisify himself that the technique is applicable as a service rather than as a research procedure. Failure to do this is as reprehensible as submitting a patient to some new surgical procedure without enquiring as to its benefit and mortality.

The final point to be emphasized is that the risk of the disorder occurring in a particular pregnancy must be estimated accurately before prenatal diagnosis is considered – in other words the consideration of prenatal diagnosis must be an integral part of genetic counselling. All too often the author has seen patients referred for prenatal diagnosis, when the risk to

Table 6.2. Some major indications for prenatal diagnosis

Advanced maternal age	Risk of affected fetus
35–40	1 in 450–100*
40+	1 in 80*
One child with neural tube defect	1 in 20–25
Parent balanced chromosomal translocation carrier	1 in 4–10
Severe, detectable autosomal or X-linked recessive metabolic disorder	1 in 4
Severe X-linked recessive disorders, not diagnosable; mother known carrier	1 in 2†

*Risk of liveborn child with Down's syndrome.
 Risk of abnormality found at amniocentesis is higher
 (*see* Chapter 4 for details).
†Chance of male pregnancy – half such males will be unaffected.

the pregnancy has not been properly evaluated, and where the risk frequently proves to be so low as to make prenatal procedures unwarranted. Even if prenatal diagnosis were free of risk (which it is not), such a slipshod approach cannot be justified. If the clinician cannot accurately evaluate the risk himself (hopefully after reading this book, he will!), then he should seek the advice of a colleague who can.

The major specific indications for prenatal diagnosis are considered individually later in this chapter, but they can be grouped into a relatively few broad categories, which are summarized in *Table* 6.2.

Approaches to Prenatal Diagnosis
A variety of techniques exists by which a prenatal diagnosis may be achieved for different disorders. At present *amniocentesis,* the procedure by which a sample of amniotic fluid and its cells is obtained from the pregnant uterus, is the technique with the widest application, and will be discussed in detail here. It is important, however, not to forget that the other approaches exist. These are summarized in *Table* 6.3 and are likely to increase steadily in importance.

The information that can be obtained from amniocentesis is illustrated

Table 6.3. Approaches to prenatal diagnosis

1. Amniocentesis
   a. Chromosomal disorders (e.g. Down's syndrome)
   b. Inherited metabolic disorders (e.g. Tay–Sachs disease)
   c. Open neural tube defects
2. Ultrasound
   a. Placental localization and exclusion of twins
   b. Anencephaly
   c. Other gross structural malformations
3. Amnioscopy (fetoscopy)
   Severe limb and other visible malformations
4. Fetal blood sampling (via amnioscope or by placental aspiration)
   a. Thalassaemias and related disorders
   b. Other severe haematological and metabolic disorders detectable
      from fetal blood
5. Maternal blood screening
   Neural tube defects

in *Fig.* 6.1. The sample should consist of clear fluid, in which are suspended the cells, fetal in origin, that can be cultured for chromosomal or biochemical studies. A bloodstained sample usually indicates damage to the placenta; a discoloured fluid may indicate fetal death, and is an important factor to note since the subsequent inevitable abortion might otherwise be attributed to the amniocentesis itself. Both situations reduce the chance of a successful cell culture.

Once obtained, the sample is usually spun immediately and duplicate cell cultures set up. The fluid can be used for alphafetoprotein estimation and, less frequently, for metabolic studies. A portion of the cell deposit may also be used for direct fetal sexing using conventional stains to detect the presence of the X chromatin or Barr body, present only in females or other individuals with more than one X chromosome. Fluorescent techniques will detect the Y chromosome of males, so that a combination of both should allow accurate sex determination in most cases. An important proviso is that the laboratory should be performing these techniques routinely; in any case, it is preferable to await the full results from cultured cells before a decision is made regarding termination.

Direct study of amniotic fluid cells has also been advocated for other disorders, e.g. open neural tube defects, where cells of neural origin may be morphologically distinguishable. Most diagnostic studies, however, whether chromosomal or biochemical, require cultured amniotic fluid cells, and depending on the numbers required, it may be 2–6 weeks before sufficient are available. It is important that cultures are checked regularly to ensure that satisfactory cell growth is occurring; if not it may be preferable to repeat amniocentesis soon, rather than to wait until it is certain that growth will not occur, by which time it may be too late.

Amniocentesis

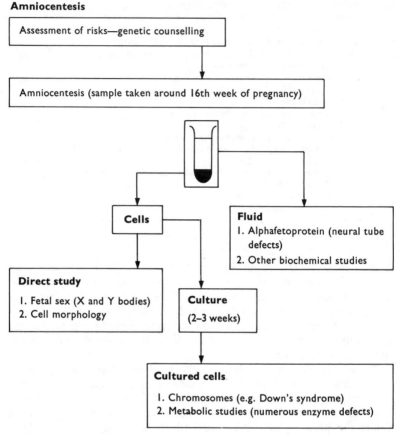

Fig. 6.1. Amniocentesis – the main steps (from Mahler and Harper, 1979, *Medicine* 10, 570).

Chromosomal Disorders

The recurrence risks for the major types of chromosome disorder have been discussed in Chapter 4, and the strength of indication for amniocentesis will depend on the magnitude of this risk as well as on the nature of the disorder and the attitude to and experience of the couple concerned in relation to it. The risks of amniocentesis will need careful consideration, especially where the risk of abnormality in the pregnancy is low. The main chromosomal indications for amniocentesis are listed in *Table* 6.4 and are considered individually here.

Advanced Maternal Age

The risk here is primarily for Down's syndrome, with a lesser risk of other trisomies. The difference in risk of a liveborn child with an abnormality

Table 6.4. Principal chromosomal indications for prenatal diagnosis (*see* Chapter 4 for detailed risk figures)

One parent carrier of a balanced autosomal translocation
Advanced maternal age
Previous child with autosomal trisomy or similar abnormality
Parent mosaic for chromosomal abnormality
Pregnancy (or male gametes) exposed to risk from irradiation or
  cytotoxic therapy (*see* Chapter 23)

and that for an abnormality found at amniocentesis, has already been emphasized (*Table* 4.5, p. 59) but there is general agreement that for women of 40 years or over, this risk is sufficient to actively ensure that all such women are informed of the risks of Down's syndrome and of the possibility of amniocentesis. Between the ages of 35 and 40 there is no general agreement as to whether such an active approach should be taken and it is likely that many women may decline amniocentesis when fully informed of the risks. Below 35 years, there is little indication for amniocentesis unless additional factors are present; the majority of women seen for amniocentesis in the 30–35 year age group have either been given an exaggerated picture of the risk for Down's syndrome or are under the impression that amniocentesis is a risk-free procedure.

Translocation Down's Syndrome (see also Chapter 4)
This rare, but high risk group makes up only 5 per cent of all cases of Down's syndrome. The risks for the offspring of balanced carriers of the various forms of translocation have been discussed in Chapter 4 and are given in *Table* 4.7, p. 62. It is clearly vital that the precise type is established from study of the index case, and that relatives at risk should be studied using blood *before* a pregnancy occurs. If the individual is a chromosomally normal sib or more distant relative there is no indication for amniocentesis. Where the parents of a child with translocation Down's syndrome are both chromosomally normal, the risk of a further affected child is also low, probably similar to that for trisomic Down's (*see below*). Although it may be reasonable to offer amniocentesis to such couples in a subsequent pregnancy, it should not be undertaken under the false assumption that the risk of Down's syndrome is high.

Trisomic Down's Syndrome and other Autosomal Trisomies (see also Chapter 4)
All studies agree that the recurrence risk is low, with the exception of very rare families where there appears to be some special factor causing clustering of chromosomal abnormalities. It is important that the chromosomes of the child, or of both parents if the child is dead are studied *before* another pregnancy is considered, and that the age of the mother is con-

sidered in estimating the recurrence risk. A risk of around twice that of the general population at an age of 35 or over is appropriate (*see* Chapter 4).

In practice most couples who have had an affected child will elect for amniocentesis in a subsequent pregnancy, even in full knowledge of the risk from the procedure and the fact that the chance of the abnormality recurring is low. Provided that they have the full facts this seems reasonable.

For other relatives of a child with trisomic Down's syndrome, there is no evidence of an increased risk in their offspring, and this should be made clear at the time of diagnosis of the index case to avoid unnecessary worry. Where such relatives remain concerned at the possibility of a chromosomal disorder in their own children, the demonstration of a normal blood karyotype is preferable to an unnecessary amniocentesis. The same approach should be employed where the index case is no longer living and no definite chromosomal status has been recognized.

Problems with Chromosomal Prenatal Diagnosis

1. Faulty diagnosis.

'Mongolism' in a relative may prove to be an entirely different disorder, and the records (or affected individual if available), should be checked wherever possible.

2. The chromosomal abnormality may be unrelated to the clinical abnormality. This is particularly seen in cases of mental retardation, where chromosome studies are commonly performed. It should especially be suspected if healthy family members show the same chromosomal pattern.

3. Normal variants.

These may be mistakenly considered to be the cause of the problem in the index case, as mentioned above, or they may be discovered in the amniotic cells of the fetus at amniocentesis. In most cases, there should be little doubt as to whether they are pathological; again help may come from finding the same pattern in a healthy parent. The findings should always be discussed with the cytogenetic laboratory that has actually performed the analysis.

4. Unrelated abnormalities.

These may be chromosomal (e.g. XXX, XXY or XYY), or a raised alpha-fetoprotein may suggest a neural tube defect in a pregnancy studied primarily for a chromosomal indication. Such findings may lead to a difficult dilemma, and in general one has to discuss the facts with the couple and respect their decision. It is always easier if the possibility of such a situation arising has been explained prior to the amniocentesis.

Neural Tube Defects [1]

The discovery that the levels of amniotic fluid alphafetoprotein are elevated in cases of open neural tube defect has provided a major advance in the avoidance of these disorders. The current situation for those pregnancies studied by amniocentesis is as follows:

Anencephaly — almost all cases detectable
Open spina bifida — 95 per cent of cases detectable
Closed spina bifida ⎫
Closed cranial defects ⎬ rarely detectable
Hydrocephalus ⎭

Because of the overlap within families between anencephaly and open and closed forms of spina bifida, a couple whose pregnancy has a normal level of alphafetoprotein cannot be guaranteed a child without a neural tube defect, but it does mean that the risk is greatly reduced. Thus where the prior risk is 1 in 20, the residual risk of an undetected neural tube defect is around 1 in 200, acceptable to most couples. The full risks are given in Chapter 10.

Before undertaking amniocentesis because of a family history of neural tube defect, the precise risk must be estimated. For first-degree relatives (risk 1 in 20 in a high incidence area such as South Wales) there is a strong case for amniocentesis, and probably also for second-degree relatives (risk 1 in 50). For third-degree relatives (first cousins), however, the risk is only around twice that of the general population (about 1 per cent in a high incidence area), so the decision may be a fine one. There seems no indication for amniocentesis where the affected individual is more distantly related.

Where the propositus has a covered spina bifida or cranial defect, amniocentesis is wise, but it is always important to point out that the procedure will not be likely to detect such a closed defect.

A question frequently asked is the risk of terminating a normal pregnancy. This will depend on the prior risk of abnormality — where this is 1 in 20 the chance of an alphafetoprotein over the 95th percentile representing a normal fetus is under 1 per cent.

Hydrocephalus is not normally detectable by amniocentesis nor (unless severe) by other measures such as ultrasound, though improved ultrasonic techniques may soon change this. Until recently it has been thought that there is no increase in incidence of anencephaly or spina bifida in families affected by hydrocephelus, except where it is secondary to a primary spinal abnormality. Analysis of pooled data[2] now suggests a small but significant risk (1 per cent) of an open neural tube defect in subsequent children, so that amniocentesis is justifiable.

Maternal Blood Screening for Neural Tube Defects

It is now clear that sensitive radioimmunoassays for alphafetoprotein in maternal blood can detect a significant proportion of open neural tube defects if undertaken at the appropriate time in pregnancy around 16—18 weeks. A number of surveys of this as a possible screening test have been and are being undertaken[3], and it is probable that widespread screening of pregnancies not at high genetic risk will soon become common, even routine practice. This has profound implications for antenatal care in general, and also means that a considerable number of women are being submitted to amniocentesis without any family history of a genetic disorder or previous awareness of the problems involved.

From the viewpoint of family members at high risk, blood screening is not an adequate substitute for amniocentesis and will merely result in delay of this; a normal serum alphafetoprotein level in a pregnancy at high prior risk should *not* stop amniocentesis being done in normal circumstances. Although there may be a case for testing maternal blood in a pregnancy where the risk is borderline (e.g. first cousins) and the couple reluctant to have amniocentesis, it must be made clear that around a quarter of the cases of spina bifida (though few of anencephaly) will be missed if reliance is placed on maternal blood alone.

Other Malformations Detectable by Raised Alphafetoprotein

Most of these have been recorded in pregnancies studied because of the risk of neural tube or chromosomal defects. *Table 6.5* summarizes some of the more important. The commonest is spontaneous intrauterine death (it

Table 6.5. Abnormalities other than neural tube defects that may cause a raised amniotic fluid AFP

Spontaneous intrauterine death
Threatened abortion
Omphalocele
Turner's syndrome
Congenital nephrosis (Finnish type)
Sacrococcygeal teratoma
Bladder exstrophy
Focal dermal hypoplasia
Meckel's syndrome

---

is important not to attribute this to the amniocentesis). Others such as omphalocele are also 'open' defects, while lymphangiomatous abnormalities are frequent in XO (Turner) pregnancies. Renal protein excretion is a special case with congenital nephrosis.

It is important to recognize that there is little information on the proportion of these abnormalities *not* detected by amniocentesis. Since they are mostly of low genetic risk anyway, they do not at present form strong indications for amniocentesis.

Some guide to the specific type of abnormality indicated by a raised amniotic fluid AFP may be given by the morphology of cells in the fluid. Abnormal cells of neural or peritoneal origin may be distinguishable from each other and from normal amniotic cells[4]. Amniotic fluid acetyl-cholinesterase levels and isoenzyme pattern may also prove helpful in this respect.

X-linked Disorders

Where a pregnancy is at high risk for an X-linked disorder, fetal sexing offers the possibility of determining whether the fetus is indeed at risk. In some cases (*Table* 6.6) direct prenatal diagnosis of an affected male is also possible. Here, fetal sexing may allow concern to be allayed in half the cases, and gives a 'fall-back' position in the event of failure of cell growth or insufficient time for complex biochemical studies.

Table 6.6. Prenatal diagnosis in X-linked disease

Feasible	
Lesch—Nyhan syndrome	
Hunter's syndrome (MPSII)	
G-6PD deficiency	
Hyperammonaemia (ornithine carbamyl transferase deficiency)	
Fabry's disease	
Haemophilia A (fetal blood required)	
Under investigation; not established	
Haemophilia B	fetal blood
Duchenne muscular dystrophy	

Where a woman is only a possible, not a definite carrier it is vital to estimate the risk before fetal sexing is undertaken and to use methods of carrier detection where applicable (*see* Chapter 5). As with any prenatal diagnostic investigation, fetal sexing should be approached as a planned procedure with the issues for and against resolved as far as possible beforehand.

Occasionally, as in haemophilia or Becker muscular dystrophy, fetal sexing may be requested for a pregnancy with an affected father, with a view to termination of a female fetus, which would inevitably be a carrier. The author has serious misgivings about the wisdom of this, since such daughters would be healthy, and since advances within the next generation are likely to allow them the option of direct prenatal diagnosis in their own future children. Sometimes eugenic grounds are given for requesting abortion of a female heterozygote; the author's personal view is that neither this nor the use of fetal sexing solely for choice of sex of the child can be justified. The development of prezygotic techniques to avoid the conception of a fetus of particular sex would be of great help in this situation and may well be achieved in the foreseeable future.

Inborn Errors of Metabolism (*see also* Chapter 20)

The development of prenatal diagnostic techniques for a variety of inborn errors of metabolism has been one of the major achievements of human biochemical genetics, even if the number of families at risk for such disorders is small in comparison with chromosomal disorders such as Down's syndrome. So many inborn errors are now prenatally detectable that this aspect is one of the first to be raised by any couple who have had an affected child. *Table* 6.7 summarizes the current situation but the list is lengthening rapidly, and will become still larger when techniques of fetal blood sampling have developed further.

Table 6.7. Prenatal diagnosis of inherited metabolic disorders (autosomal recessive inheritance unless indicated) (unless otherwise indicated, the diagnosis is made from cultured amniotic fluid cells)

Disorder	Usual enzyme deficiency	Prenatal diagnosis	Comments
Acid phosphatase deficiency (lysosomal)	Acid phosphatase	Made	
Adenosine deaminase deficiency (combined immuno-deficiency)	Adenosine deaminase	Made	
Adrenogenital syndrome	21-Hydroxylase	Made	Amniotic fluid analysis; also indirectly by HLA linkage
Argininosuccinic aciduria	Argininosuccinase	Made	Argininosuccinic acid also raised in amniotic fluid
Citrullinaemia	Argininosuccinate synthetase	Possible	
Cystathioninuria	Cystathionase	Possible	Probably a harmless anomaly
Cystinosis	Unknown	Made	Accumulation of intra-cellular S^{35} labelled cystine used
Fabry's disease	α-galactosidase	Made	X-linked; variable expression
Farber's disease	Ceramidase	Made	
Fucosidosis	α-L-fucosidase	Possible	
Galactosaemia (classic)	Galactose-1-phosphate uridyl transferase	Made	Treatment available (*see* p. 79)
Galactosaemia (galactokinase deficiency)	Galactokinase	Possible	Relatively benign and treatable disorder
Gaucher's disease	Glucocerebrosidase	Made	Heterogeneous
Generalized ganglio-sidosis	β-galactosidase	Made	
Glucose-6-phosphate dehydrogenase deficiency	G-6PD	Possible	Often mild. Many enzyme variants. X-linked
Glycogenosis Type II (Pompe's disease)	α-1,4-glucosidase	Made	Heterogeneous
Glycogenosis Type III	Amylo 1-6-glucosidase	Possible	
Haemoglobin S disease	β chain substitution	Made	Severity variable. Fetal blood required (but *see also* p. 92)

Disorder	Usual enzyme deficiency	Prenatal diagnosis	Comments
Haemophilia A	Factor VIII (CAG)	Made	Pure fetal serum required. X-linked
Haemophilia B	Factor IX	Possible	Fetal blood required. X-linked
Homocystinuria	Cystathionine synthetase	Possible	Heterogeneous
Hyperammonaemia, X-linked	Ornithine carbamyl transferase	Possible	X-linked; variable expression in female
Hypercholesterol-aemia, familial	Low-density lipo-protein receptors	Made	Homozygote only detectable
Hypophosphatasia	Alkaline phosphatase	Possible	Only severe infantile type detectable
'I' cell disease (mucolipidosis II)	? Lysosomal membrane defect	Made	Increase in multiple lysosomal enzymes
Krabbe's disease	β-galactosidase	Made	
Lesch–Nyhan syndrome	Hypoxanthine-guanine-phosphoribosyl-transferase	Made	X-linked recessive. Heterogeneous
Mannosidosis	α-mannosidase	Possible	
Maple syrup urine disease	α-ketoacid decarboxylase	Made	
Metachromatic leucodystrophy	Arylsulphatase A	Made	Heterogeneous
Methylmalonic aciduria	Methylmalonyl CO A mutase	Made	Methylmalonic acid detectable in amniotic fluid. May be treatable *in utero.* Heterogeneous
Mucopoly-saccharidosis I (Hurler's syndrome)	α-L-iduronidase	Made	MPS Is (Scheie syndrome) has same enzyme deficient
Mucopoly-saccharidosis II (Hunter's syndrome)	Iduronate sulphatase	Made	X-linked; enzymatic diagnosis possible from amniotic fluid as well as cells
Mucopoly-saccharidosis III A (Sanfilippo A syndrome)	Heparan sulphate sulphatase	Made	
Mucopoly-saccharidosis III B (Sanfilippo B syndrome)	α-N-acetyl-hexosaminidase	Possible	Carrier detection feasible on serum
Mucopoly-saccharidosis IV (Morquio's syndrome)	Chondroitin sulphate sulphatase	Potentially possible	
Mucopoly-saccharidosis VI (Maroteaux-Lamy syndrome)	Aryl sulphatase B	Possible	

Disorder	Usual enzyme deficiency	Prenatal diagnosis	Comments
Niemann–Pick disease	Sphingomyelinase	Made	Heterogeneous
Porphyria, acute intermittent	Uroporphyrinogen synthetase	Made	Autosomal dominant
Porphyria, congenital erythropoietic	Uroporphyrinogen cosynthetase	Possible	
Propionic acidaemia	Propionyl CO A carboxylase	Made	Also directly detectable from amniotic fluid
Refsum's disease	Phytanic acid oxidase	Possible	
Sandhoff's disease	β-N-acetyl hexosaminidase (A and B)	Made	
Thalassaemia (β)	Defective β chain synthesis	Made	Fetal blood required (but see also Chapter 21)
Tay–Sachs disease	β-N-Acetyl hexosaminidase A	Made	Carrier detection and high risk population screening feasible
Wolman's disease	Acid lipase	Possible	
Xeroderma pigmentosum	DNA repair enzyme (endonuclease)	Made	Heterogeneous

The following points need consideration when the prenatal diagnosis of a metabolic disorder is being considered.

1. The great majority of these disorders follow autosomal recessive inheritance, so that only sibs of affected patients are at high (1 in 4) risk. Risks for other relatives are rarely high enough to warrant undertaking prenatal diagnosis.

2. Most disorders require cultured amniotic cells for their diagnosis; in general if a particular enzyme defect can be detected in the cultured skin fibroblast it can also be detected in cultured amniotic cells.

3. Large numbers of cells are often required, adding delay and uncertainty which should be explained beforehand. A late termination may be unacceptable to a couple who would accept termination in early pregnancy. Techniques utilizing very small numbers of cells have yet to prove their reliability.

4. Many of the techniques are exceptionally difficult and can only be undertaken by a very few laboratories. Careful advance planning is essential since cells may have to be sent long distances. Fortunately, a remarkable degree of cooperation exists between laboratories involved in this work, and there are several updated lists of centres with experience in different disorders (see p. 272). Careful distinction is needed between a centre that is 'interested' in a disorder and one that has proven experience in its prenatal diagnosis.

5. Wherever possible samples from the affected individual should be studied alongside those at risk. If the affected child is likely to die every effort should be made to reach a precise enzymatic diagnosis beforehand, and to arrange for storage of cultured cells or post-mortem material to be used at a later date. Failure to do this may result in serious problems in relation to a future pregnancy.

A few inherited metabolic diseases can be diagnosed directly from amniotic fluid itself, though the use of cultured cells is usually desirable as a back up. These include the organic acidurias (propionic and methylmalonic aciduria), mycopolysaccharidosis II (Hunter's syndrome) the 21-hydroxylase form of congenital adrenal hyperplasia, and congenital nephrosis (by elevated amniotic alphafetoprotein).

Another group that is important to distinguish is the group of disorders that at present *cannot* be recognized prenatally. This includes cystic fibrosis, phenylketonuria (for which newborn screening is available), type I glycogenosis (where, like phenylketonuria, the enzyme defect is localized to the liver) and some others, listed in *Table* 6.8. At present the commoner non-Mendelian metabolic disorders, such as congenital hypothyroidism, diabetes and other endocrine deficiencies are not diagnosable *in utero*.

Table 6.8. Some major inborn errors of metabolism *not* at present detectable prenatally

Cystic fibrosis
Phenylketonuria
Alkaptonuria
Glycogenosis type I
Tyrosinosis
Histidinaemia
Hereditary fructose intolerance

Prenatal Prediction by Genetic Linkage

If the locus for a particular disease is known to be closely linked to that for a genetic marker such as a blood group or similar polymorphism, it may be possible to predict from the marker phenotype whether an individual also has inherited the gene for the disease. Since most markers are expressed independent of age, such a prediction should be valid in early childhood and also — if the marker can be detected — in antenatal life.

With the rapid development of our understanding of the human gene map in recent years this approach holds out considerable promise for the numerous disorders where we either do not know the underlying biochemical defect, or where it is not expressed in cultured cells. *Table* 6.9 shows some of the potentially useful linkages; their number is likely to increase steadily.

Table 6.9. Prenatal prediction by genetic linkage. Some potential applications

Disease	Marker locus
Myotonic dystrophy	Secretor
Haemophilia A	G-6PD
Congenital adrenal hyperplasia ⎫ Spinocerebellar ataxia (one type) ⎰	HLA
Congenital cataract (one type)	Duffy blood group
Sickle-cell disease	Linked DNA sequence

In practice the use of linkage in this way is extremely limited at present, for a number of reasons:

1. The entire family must be studied and relevant members may be dead or unavailable

2. Most loci (except HLA) are not polymorphic enough to allow more than a small proportion of families to be studied.

3. Depending on the closeness of linkage there will be a definite error rate in prediction because of crossing over.

4. Genetic heterogeneity may confuse the situation.

Myotonic dystrophy[5] and haemophilia[6] are two disorders where linkage has actually been used in prenatal prediction, but in the latter this approach has already been superseded by direct prenatal diagnosis from fetal blood.

A recent exciting development has been the use of DNA polymorphisms, such as that occurring close to the haemoglobin β chain locus. This has been used to diagnose sickle-cell disease[7] (*see* Chapter 21) and has the great advantage of requiring only a small bumber of uncultured amniotic fluid cells, not fetal blood. As our knowledge of DNA structure at other loci increases this approach will become applicable to other Mendelian disorders and will be of particular importance in allowing detection of those numerous conditions where the primary defect is either unknown or undetectable in cultured cells.

Amniocentesis
Practical Aspects
It is important that clinicians referring patients for amniocentesis or suggesting its application should realize what is involved and how best to utilize the service that is provided. The need for proper assessment and genetic counselling *before* a pregnancy is undertaken has already been stressed, but several points are often overlooked.

1. *Timing.* 15—16 weeks' gestation is the earliest that a satisfactory sample can reliably be obtained, so the couple must be prepared to accept a termination at 18 weeks or sometimes later. It is not uncommon for a

patient's attitude to change during pregnancy, particularly once fetal movement has occurred.

2. *Who should perform the procedure?* There is little doubt that the risks are increased if amniocentesis is done by an 'occasional operator' and there is much to be said for a centralized service in which skilled amniocentesis, accurate genetic counselling and appropriate laboratory facilities can all be combined.

3. *The procedure itself.* Some patients expect amniocentesis to be a frightening and painful procedure, which it is not. Direct needling after ultrasound scan has localized the placenta and confirmed the correct gestation can be done under local anaesthesia without need for hospital admission, though rest for 2 hours afterwards is advisable. It is surprising how many women are referred without a clear picture having been given of what amniocentesis entails; the author holds a clinic jointly with the obstetricians involved which allows a careful explanation of the procedure and its risks as well as ensuring that correct genetic counselling has been given.

4. *Results and follow-up.* The couple must be warned that a result may take up to 3 weeks (sometimes longer for biochemical studies) and that there is a possibility that a repeat sample may be needed. The possibility of abnormality unrelated to that primarily being looked for should be mentioned (e.g. a neural tube defect in a pregnancy at risk for Down's syndrome) and a clear policy must be defined in the event of no definite answer being reached because of culture failure or other reasons. Follow-up after delivery is important not only to check the correctness of the prediction, but because the outcome may affect the genetic risk to subsequent pregnancies.

The Risks of Amniocentesis

It is only recently that these have become clearly defined, as a result of the publication of several large studies. The study giving most extensive information has been one of 2400 pregnancies requiring amniocentesis, carried out in Britain by the Medical Research Council[8], specifically investigating the risks. Others from USA[9] and Canada[10] have shown lower risks but were not so specifically designed to assess this aspect. The true risks may be somewhere in between. Taking the MRC study as the basis, the following figures seem appropriate as representing the upper limits of risk.

1. *Abortion.* There is an added risk of 1–1·5 per cent due to the procedure (2·9 per cent compared with 1·6 per cent in the control series). Repeat amniocentesis carries a much higher risk of abortion (9 per cent).

2. *Perinatal problems.* There appears to be a threefold increase of neonatal respiratory distress, occurring in around 3 per cent of offspring, and an increased incidence of postural orthopaedic abnormalities (in particular talipes and congenital dislocation of the hip) occurring in

around 2·4 per cent. Overall there is an increase of almost 1 per cent in perinatal mortality. Apart from these major considerations there is a slightly increased risk of rhesus sensitization, and possibly an increased rate of antepartum haemorrhage, though there is some dispute over this last possibility. Maternal risks are minimal.

These risk figures make it quite clear that amniocentesis, like any other invasive procedure, carries a definite mortality and morbidity for the fetus, and make it essential that it is used selectively and appropriately, as well as for the risks to be carefully explained to these couples who may be considering it.

Other Approaches to Prenatal Diagnosis
Ultrasound[11]
The principal use of ultrasound at present is ancillary to amniocentesis in locating the placenta, establishing an accurate gestational date and excluding multiple pregnancy and fetal death. It allows recognition of anencephaly in most cases, and will detect some (but not all) cases of spina bifida. It is likely that other structural malformations such as congenital

Table 6.10. Use of diagnostic ultrasound in early pregnancy

Dating of pregnancy
Placental localization
Multiple pregnancy
Hydatidiform mole or blighted ovum
Anencephaly
Spina bifida ⎱
Microcephaly ⎬ some cases only
Hydrocephalus ⎰
Polycystic kidneys (severe infantile type)
Severe short limbed dwarfism and other limb defects

heart defects, may in future become detectable by ultrasound, but at present congenital polycystic kidney disease is the only disorder where experience is sufficient to rely on the technique; even here it is likely only to be of help in cases with gross renal enlargement at birth, which show a close degree of concordance among sibs (see Chapter 18). Table 6.10 summarizes the current position. It must be emphasized that there is a considerable difference between the sensitivity and accuracy of ultrasound in the hands of an experienced operator with modern equipment and that available in most general hospitals.

Fetoscopy (Amnioscopy)
The development of small calibre flexible fibreoptic instruments that can be inserted into the amniotic cavity under local anaesthesia (usually with

sedation in addition) makes direct inspection of the fetus between 18–22 weeks' gestation a real possibility. In particular, malformations involving the limbs (especially digits), face (including defects of the ear and clefting) and genitals can be recognized or excluded. The spine is less easy to inspect. The risk of fetoscopy by the few experienced operators is still high (5–10 per cent risk of abortion). Continued leakage of amniotic fluid may occur. Thus at present, the main indication is in recessively inherited severe limb and craniofacial defects where the abnormality is sufficiently constant to be excluded by a normal fetoscopy. Dominantly inherited defects where one parent is affected are a less definite indication – not only does there tend to be greater variation in phenotype, but the disorders are milder and often amenable to surgical correction. It is likely that the criteria for fetoscopy will soon become clearer as its scope, risks and limitations become better defined.

Fetoscopic skin biopsy has recently been used to diagnose the letalis form of epidermolysis bullosa prenatally (*see* p. 183).

Fetal Blood Sampling[12]

A fetal blood sample may be obtained by placental aspiration or under direct vision. In the former case it will be mixed with maternal blood, and techniques to separate fetal red blood cells may be required before the

Table 6.11. Prenatal diagnosis from fetal blood sample

Proven applications
Thalassaemias
Sickle-cell disease
Haemophilia A
Probable applications
Chromosomal instability syndromes (e.g. Fanconi anaemia)
Haemophilia B
Red-cell enzyme defects
Blood groups
Potential applications
Duchenne muscular dystrophy
Immune deficiency disorders

sample can be used. Direct sampling requires fetoscopy, with blood being aspirated from a vessel on the placental surface or from the root of the cord; here the contamination is likely to be with amniotic fluid rather than maternal blood.

Both techniques carry a considerable risk (up to 10 per cent) of inducing abortion, but this is declining with more experience and already there are clinical indications for the procedure being used as a service rather than on an experimental basis. These are listed in *Table* 6.11, together with some likely future applications. The thalassaemias are the principal indication at present[13], and the technique is already proving valuable in communities with a high incidence of β-thalassaemia, where pregnancies at high risk can be identified by carrier studies on the parents. It is likely that other severe red cell disorders, both haemoglobinopathies and enzyme defects, will become detectable, though whether this approach will prove acceptable in the third world countries where they form a major problem remains to be seen. Fetal blood group determination may prove to be helpful when more close genetic linkages with serious diseases are established.

Obtaining a satisfactory fetal serum sample is much more of a problem than obtaining fetal red cells. The most important application at present appears to be in the detection of haemophilia A, where the procoagulant Factor VIII activity is absent in fetal serum, and where prenatal diagnosis is now feasible[14, 15]. The use of fetal creatine kinase for the detection of Duchenne muscular dystrophy has also been attempted, but our lack of information as to the range of this enzyme in the affected fetus makes this uncertain at present (*see* Chapter 9) and cases are now known to have been missed. It seems likely that immune deficiency disorders may also become suitable for diagnosis from fetal serum.

As with any rapidly developing techniques, the clinician must be clear on which indications are firm ones and which are still experimental, and be prepared to protect his patients from hasty and over-enthusiastic application of a technique which may still be carrying considerable risk and margin of error.

Before raising the possibility of this procedure with a couple it is essential that the clinician concerned should:

a. Make sure that the pregnancy or intended pregnancy is indeed at high risk.

b. That fetoscopy has indeed been established for the particular condition.

c. That he has personally discussed the problem with a unit that has the necessary technical and laboratory expertise.

Twins and Prenatal Diagnosis

The discovery of a twin pregnancy poses obvious practical problems in undertaking amniocentesis, but it also alters the genetic risk figures that would normally be given for a singleton pregnancy. The problems involved in estimating the modified risks have recently been discussed by Hunter and Cox[16], and are summarized in *Table* 6.12. It is assumed here that 1/3 of twin pairs are monozygous.

It can be seen that in general the risks are considerably higher than for a singleton pregnancy and that they are altered if information is available on one twin from amniocentesis. Clearly the couple concerned should be

Table 6.12. Genetic risks in twin pregnancies (after Hunter and Cox, 1979)

	Chromosome abnormality	Neural tube defect	X-linked (fetal sexing only)	X-linked (specific diagnostic test)	Autosomal recessive
Before amniocentesis					
Risk for singleton pregnancy	Y*	1/25	1/2	1/4	1/4
Risk for at least one twin being affected	5/3 Y	2/25	2/3	3/8	3/8
Risk of both twins being affected	≃1/3 Y	<1/100	1/3	1/8	1/8
Twin A normal risk of twin B being abnormal	2/3 Y	1/25	1/3	1/6	1/6
After amniocentesis (not one sac successfully tested)					
Twin A abnormal chance of twin B being normal	2/3 − 2/3 Y	9/10	1/3	1/2	1/2
Twin A abnormal risk of twin B being abnormal	1/3 + 2/3 Y	1/10	2/3	1/2	1/2

*Risk will vary with maternal age, etc.

informed of these altered risks, and the same is true even when prenatal diagnosis is not being considered.

A further point to be considered is that the normal range of maternal serum alphafetoprotein is raised in twin pregnancies.

Example

A 37-year-old woman whose sister had suffered from spina bifida was found on ultrasonography to be carrying twins in her third pregnancy. The chance of at least one twin having a neural tube defect was estimated as 1 in 25 (twice the risk for a singleton pregnancy), while the risk for Down's syndrome was estimated as 1 in 150 (5/3 the risk for a singleton pregnancy).

Serum alphafetoprotein was at the 98th percentile for a singleton pregnancy but amniocentesis was impossible because of a large single anterior placenta. Ultrasonography of the fetal spines was normal. Healthy twin boys were subsequently born.

References
1. UK Collaborative Study on alphafetoprotein in relation to neural-tube defects (1977) *Lancet* **1**, 1323–1332.
2. Cohen T., Stern E. and Rosenmann A. (1979) Sib risk of neural tube defect: is prenatal diagnosis indicated following the birth of a hydrocephalic child? *J. Med. Genet.* **16**, 14–16.

3. Ferguson-Smith M. A., Rawlinson H. A., May H. M. et al. (1978) Avoidance of anencephalic and spina bifida births by maternal serum-alpha-fetoprotein screening. *Lancet* 1, 1330–1333.
4. Gosden C. and Brock D. J. H. (1978) Amniotic fluid cell morphology in early antenatal prediction of abortion and low birth weight. *Br. Med. J.* 2, 1186–1189.
5. Insley J., Bird G. W. G., Harper P. S. et al. (1976) Prenatal prediction of myotonic dystrophy. *Lancet* 1, 806.
6. Edgell C. J. S., Kirkman H. N., Clemons E. et al. (1978) Prenatal diagnosis by linkage: hemophilia A and polymorphic glucose-6-phosphate dehydrogenase. *Am. J. Hum. Genet.* 30, 80–84.
7. Kan Y. W. and Dozy A. (1978) Antenatal diagnosis of sickle cell anaemia by DNA analysis of amniotic fluid cells. *Lancet* 2, 910–912.
8. Medical Research Council Working Party on Amniocentesis (1978) An assessment of the hazards of amniocentesis. *Br. J. Obstet. Gynaecol.* 85, Suppl. 2, 1–41.
9. United States Institute of Child Health and Human Development Study Group (1976) *JAMA* 236, 1471–1476.
10. Simpson N. E., Dallaire L., Miller J. R. et al. (1976) Prenatal diagnosis of genetic disease in Canada: report of a collaborative study. *Canad. Med. Assoc. J.* 115, 739–748.
11. Donald I. (1978) Ultrasonography in the diagnosis of fetal malformations. In: Scrimgeour J. B. (ed.), *Towards the Prevention of Fetal Malformation.* Edinburgh University Press, pp. 123–137.
12. Rodeck C. H. and Campbell S. (1978) Sampling pure fetal blood by fetoscopy in second trimester of pregnancy. *Br. Med. J.* 2, 728–730.
13. Huehns E. R. (1979) Antenatal diagnosis in beta thalassaemia. *Advanced Medicine* 15, 259–266.
14. Peake I. R. and Bloom A. L. (1978) Immunoradiometric assay of procoagulant factor VIII antigen in plasma and serum and its reduction in haemophilia. *Lancet* 1, 473–475.
15. Mibashan R. S., Rodeck C. H., Thumpston J. K. et al. (1979) Plasma assay of fetal factor VIIIC and IX for prenatal diagnosis of haemophilia. *Lancet* 1, 1309–1311.
16. Hunter A. G. W. and Cox D. M. (1979) Counseling problems when twins are discovered at genetic amniocentesis. *Clin. Genet.* 16, 34–42.

Further Reading

Murken J. D., Stengel-Rutkowski S. and Schwinger E. (ed.) (1979) *Prenatal Diagnosis.* Proceedings of the 3rd European Conference on Prenatal Diagnosis of Genetic Disorders. Stuttgart, Enke.
Scrimgeour J. (ed.) (1978) *Towards the Prevention of Fetal Abnormality.* Edinburgh University Press.
Siggers D. (1978) *Prenatal Diagnosis of Genetic Disease.* Oxford, Blackwell. A brief but clear introduction.
Wald N. J. and Cuckle H. S. (1980) Alphafetoprotein in the antenatal diagnosis of open neural tube defects. *Br. J. Hosp. Med.* 23, 473–489.

CHAPTER SEVEN

Special Problems in Genetic Counselling

Consanguinity

Consanguinity, or marriage between close relatives, is a common and important problem in genetic counselling. Where an inherited disorder is present in the family, consanguinity may significantly influence the risks, while even without a known disorder couples who are closely related may be concerned about the risks to their offspring.

There are three aspects of consanguinity which need to be considered in relation to genetic counselling.

1. What is the exact relationship of the two individuals?
2. How is the risk of a genetic disorder in the family influenced by the occurrence of consanguinity?
3. How likely is it that any harmful gene might be handed by both members of the couple to a child, i.e. that the child is homozygous by descent for that gene?

An attempt is made here to answer these questions in simple terms, avoiding a complex mathematical approach. These same questions are of more general interest to population geneticists, and detailed accounts of the subject can be found in genetics textbooks.

Genetic Relationships

An accurate idea of how individuals are related is essential in all genetic counselling, regardless of the presence or absence of consanguinity, but when a marriage between close relatives is being considered, it becomes particularly important. *Table* 7.1 summarizes the main categories of relationship, and it is always important to construct a precise pedigree pattern rather than to rely on verbal descriptions, which may be confusing. *Table* 7.2 gives examples.

Marriage between first-degree relatives is almost universally prohibited by law and social custom, but incestuous relationships, usually between father and daughter or between sibs, are considerably commoner than is generally recognized, and give rise to particular problems discussed below. Marriage between second-degree relatives is also legally barred in many countries, though uncle—niece marriage is frequent in some Asian communities.

First cousin marriages are the most common reason for couples seeking

Table 7.1. Degrees of relationship

	Proportion of genes shared
First degree	
Sibs	
Dizygotic twins	1/2
Parents	
Children	
Second degree	
Half sibs	
Uncles, aunts	1/4
Nephews, nieces	
Third degree	
First cousins	
Half uncles, aunts	1/8
Half nephews, nieces	

genetic advice; these are legal in many Western countries, but may be the subject of religious or social restrictions. In many Asian communities they are actively encouraged. The less common half uncle—niece marriage shown in *Table* 7.2 is in genetic terms identical to a first cousin marriage.

Among the more distant relationships the problem of terminology may cause confusion. The term 'removed' refers to a difference in generations between the individuals — thus the son of one's first cousin is a first cousin once removed while the children of one's parents' first cousins are one's second cousins.

It should be noted that the 'degrees' of relationship shown in *Table* 7.1 are those used in genetic terminology, and also in English canon and common law, but *not* in civil law, where a different approach is used. Thus, uncle and niece, who would generally be considered second-degree relatives, would be termed 'third-degree relatives' in civil law.

Some of the legal aspects of consanguineous marriages are given in *Table* 7.3. It is helpful in genetic counselling to be aware of these since many couples have unspoken fears about the legality of a relationship as well as the genetic risks. Clearly the situation will vary between countries, and in the USA between individual states. Farrow and Juberg[1] have summarized the confusing situation for the USA, which provides some remarkable inconsistencies: thus first cousin marriages are illegal in over half the states, while half niece or half nephew marriages are prohibited in only a quarter of states. Some states prohibit marriages between first cousins once removed. On the other hand eleven states allow marriages between half sibs.

Quite apart from these complexities, there are a number of restrictions on marriages between *unrelated* indiviudals. Thus, the wife of an uncle may be considered as a legal aunt even though no genetic relationship

Table 7.2. Patterns of relationship

Relationship (between shaded individuals)	Degree of relationship	Proportion of genes shared	Chance of homozygosity by descent (F)
Monozygotic twins	–	1	–
Dizygotic twins	First	1/2	1/4
Sibs	First	1/2	1/4
Parent–child	First	1/2	1/4
Uncle (aunt) – niece (nephew)	Second	1/4	1/8
Half sibs	Second	1/4	1/8
Double first cousins		1/4	1/8
First cousins	Third	1/8	1/16
Half uncle niece (or similar combination)	Third	1/8	1/16
First cousins once removed	Fourth	1/16	1/32
Second cousins	Fifth	1/32	1/64

Relationship (between shaded individuals)	Degree of relationship	Proportion of genes shared	Chance of homozygosity by descent (F)
Second cousins once removed		1/64	1/128
Third cousins		1/128	1/256

Table 7.3. Legal restrictions on marriage (UK and USA)

Marriage	UK	USA
Full sibs	Illegal	Illegal (all states)
Parent—child	Illegal	Illegal
Grandparent—grandchild	Illegal	Illegal
Half sibs	Illegal	Illegal in 42 states
Uncle (aunt)—niece (nephew)	Illegal	Illegal
Half uncle—niece (or half aunt—nephew)	Illegal	Illegal in 18 states
First cousins	Legal	Illegal in 30 states
First cousin once removed	Legal	Illegal in 7 states
Double first cousin	Legal	Illegal in N. Carolina

exists. In addition, different religions may have specific prohibitions over and above the legal requirement.

Taking all these facts together, it can be seen that there are numerous legal as well as genetic pitfalls confronting those involved in genetic counselling for consanguineous marriages; if there is any doubt, the couple should obtain legal advice and this aspect should be clarified before the genetic risks are discussed in detail.

Risks of Consanguinity with a Specific Genetic Disorder in the Family
In general, consanguinity will have no effect on risks if the disorder is X-linked recessive or autosomal dominant, unless both of the couple concerned actually have the condition or carry the gene concerned.

Autosomal recessive inheritance provides the main problem; it is likely that risks are also increased for polygenic disorders, even though this is difficult to estimate.

The essential question to be asked for an autosomal recessive disorder is − what is the chance that the harmful gene will have passed down both sides of the family simultaneously and appear in homozygous state in the child? The situation is best dealt with by the example shown in *Fig.* 7.1.

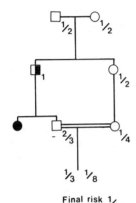

Fig. 7.1. Genetic risks in a consanguineous marriage (*see* text for explanation).

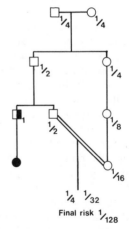

Fig. 7.2. Genetic risks in a consanguineous marriage (first cousins once removed). The chance of a child being homozygous for (i.e. affected by) the rare autosomal recessive disorder present in the husband's niece is 1 in 128.

Here, a man having a sister with a rare autosomal recessive disorder has married his first cousin. We can ignore the very small added risk of mutation or the gene being present by chance.

The chance of the husband carrying the harmful gene is 2/3 (*not* 2/4, as is commonly thought, since the homozygous affected category has been excluded). The chance of a child receiving the gene from him is thus 1/3.

The chance of the wife (first cousin) also being a carrier must now be estimated. Both parents of the husband must be carriers and one of the common paternal grandparents also must be, so the chance of their daughter being a carrier is 1/2 and for their grand-daughter (the wife in the couple being considered) 1/4. The chance of the gene being transmitted to her child will be 1/8.

The risk of the child receiving the gene from both sides simultaneously, i.e. of having the disorder, is simply the product: $1/3 \times 1/8 = 1/24$.

A second example is given in *Fig.* 7.2 which is a little more complex, but the approach is the same. Every generation added to the path diminishes the risk by one-half.

General Risks of Consanguinity

Estimates of risk for the offspring of consanguineous marriages when no disorder is known in the family are based on two approaches — information on the probable number of deleterious recessive genes carried by healthy individuals in the population, and surveys of the outcome of pregnancies from consanguineous marriages.

Several studies have suggested that everyone carries at least one gene for a harmful recessive disorder, and probably at least two for lethal conditions that would result in a spontaneous abortion or stillbirth. Using this as a basis, risks can easily be estimated if one knows the relationship of the couple concerned.

The simplest approach is to trace the fate of such a harmful gene from the common ancestor or ancestors to the offspring at risk, in a manner similar to that described in the previous section. *Fig.* 7.3 shows this for a first cousin marriage, where it is clear that the risk of one harmful recessive gene reaching the offspring by both sides simultaneously is 1 in 64. Since the other common ancestor has to be considered as well, the total risk is 1 in 32. If the two lethal genes carried by each individual are considered in the same way, the risk is 1 in 16. This latter estimate is identical to the risk of *any* gene being homozygous by descent in the offspring, a figure known as the coefficient of consanguinity (F); this forms the generally used yardstick for measuring closeness of relationship between two individuals (*Table* 7.1) and can also be used in connection with populations as well as individuals as discussed below.

Studies of the actual empiric risks to the offspring of consanguineous marriages summarized in *Table* 7.4, vary considerably between populations.

It is difficult also to separate any increase in specific genetic disorders from problems with a large environmental contribution. Thus, in the extensive study of Schull[2] in Japan, the offspring of first cousin marriages followed over a 10-year period showed a 3 per cent increase in mortality over those with unrelated parents, but only a small increase in severe malformations (1·7 per cent compared with 1·0 per cent). Offspring

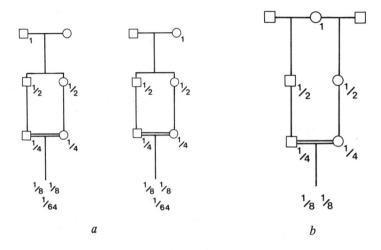

Fig. 7.3. *a,* First cousin marriage. The chance of a harmful gene in a common ancestor being homozygous by descent in the child is 1 in 64. Since there are two common ancestors the risk will be twice this (total risk 1 in 32). *b,* Marriage between half first cousins. The situation is as for full first cousins but there is only one common ancestor to be considered (total risk 1 in 64).

Table 7.4. Observed increase in severe abnormalities and mortality among offspring of consanguineous parents

Incestuous matings	30%
First cousins	3%
First cousins once removed and second cousins	1%

of first cousin once removed and second cousin marriages showed no increase in malformation rate.

Studies of the offspring of incestuous matings[3, 4, 5, 6] have confirmed the high predicted risk to offspring, and show a risk of around 1/3 of childhood death or severe abnormality. In addition, there appears to be an increased risk of mental retardation without physical abnormality, so that only about half of such children may be fully normal. This poses a special problem since such children are commonly placed for adoption, and adoption agencies and potential adoptive parents will want to know how great is the risk of an undetected serious recessive disorder. It seems likely that around three-quarters of such disorders will express themselves in the first 6 months of life, so it is probably reasonable to wait until around this age before finalizing an adoption placement. It is also worth actively testing for the commoner autosomal recessive disorders such as cystic fibrosis and phenylketonuria.

There is no clear evidence for a significant effect of consanguinity on intelligence in first cousin or more distantly related marriages.

In summary, consanguinity without known genetic disease in the family appears to cause an increase in mortality and malformation rate which is extremely marked in the children of incestuous matings, but which is of little significance when the relationship is more distant than first cousins. First cousin marriages, the most common counselling problem, seem to have an added risk of about 3 per cent, so that a total risk of 5 per cent for abnormality or death in early childhood, about double the general population risk, is a reasonable though approximate guide. It seems likely that the risk is less for populations with a long tradition of cousin marriage; recent studies in India have shown no clear difference in malformations or perinatal loss between a consanguineous and non-consanguineous group.

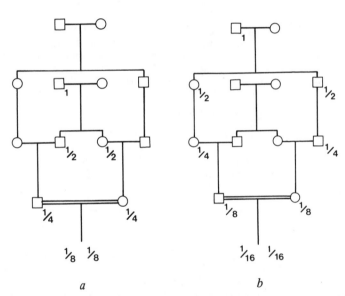

Fig. 7.4. Estimation of risks with multiple consanguinity. One harmful recessive allele is assumed for each individual. *a*, Risk = 2 × 1/8 × 1/8 = 1/32. *b*, Risk = 2 × 1/16 × 1/16 = 1/128. Total risk = 1/32 + 1/128 = 5/128 (≙ 4 per cent).

Multiple Consanguinity

Individuals may be related to each other in more than one way. This causes difficulty in drawing the pedigree as well as in calculating the precise degree of relationship. The simplest approach is to deal with each mode of relationship separately, work out the coefficient of consanguinity for each, and then add them. More complex situations may need the help of a colleague expert in population genetics, but this method should be sufficient for most counselling situations. *Fig.* 7.4 gives an example.

The couple are first cousins by one set of parents, but also second cousins by the other set. Their coefficient of consanguinity (F) is thus that for first cousins (1/16) + that for second cousins (1/64) giving a total of 5/64. The risk of a serious recessive disorder assuming one harmful recessive gene per person would be about half this, i.e. 5/128 or about 4 per cent.

Alternatively, the route of a harmful gene can be plotted as in *Fig.* 7.4 taking the 'inner loop' (first cousin) first and then the outer (second cousin loop). The two pathways give risks of 1/32 and 1/128 respectively (each path must be gone over twice for the two common ancestors), giving a combined risk of 5/128, as did the first approach.

Inbred Populations

It is possible for a couple to be closely related simply because they are both members of an inbred population which has many of its genes in common.

Such populations, particularly when isolated or derived from a small founding population, are often notable for the rare recessively inherited diseases occurring in them[7] and for many of them estimates of the coefficient of consanguinity (F) for the population as a whole are available. Even in the most inbred the level of consanguinity rarely approaches the first cousin level.

In some cases the frequency of carriers of a harmful gene in the population may be known, and this may be used in counselling. Thus, for a healthy man whose sister had Tay—Sachs disease, the risk of marrying a carrier would be 1 in 20 if he married someone of Ashkenazi Jewish descent, but only 1 in 400 if he married a non-Jewish person.

In the absence of such information the risks are similar to where the partners are known relatives with a particular coefficient of consanguinity. Thus a couple from the highly inbred Canadian Hutterite community (F = 0·03 or 1/67) would be predicted to have a risk of recessively inherited disorders in the offspring similar to that of second cousins (F = 1/64). Practical proof of these risks is rarely available however.

Where a known consanguineous marriage occurs in an already inbred population, the two contributions must be added. Thus the risk of homozygosity by descent (= F) for a first cousin marriage in a Welsh Gypsy population[8] would be:

1/16 (F for first cousin marriage)
+ 1/50 (F for whole population)
= 1/12
The risk for a serious recessive disorder would be half this = 1/24 (as discussed above).

Paternity and Non-paternity

The uncertainty of paternity is a subject that has always concerned people, more for legal and social reasons than for any connections with genetic disease. Indeed, some societies in the past have not recognized the existence of paternity at all, while only in comparatively recent times has it been accepted that the paternal and maternal contributions to the child are approximately equal. The possibility of non-paternity must always be considered when trying to explain a puzzling pedigree pattern; non-maternity by contrast is an exceptionally rare problem; it is seen chiefly in possible confused identity of infants in maternity hospitals and in instances where a woman claims a kidnapped baby to be her own.

The testing of paternity depends almost entirely on the use of genetic polymorphisms detectable in blood; clearly the more polymorphic a system is, the greater is the chance of it distinguishing between two individuals, which is the object of the exercise. The main systems are:

1. Blood group antigens (especially ABO, Rh, MNS, Duffy, Kidd).
2. Red cell enzymes (especially acid phosphatase, PGM, GPT).
3. Serum proteins (especially haptoglobins, GM, Gc).
4. HLA antigens.

Haemoglobin variants, such as HbS, may be helpful in ethnic groups where their frequency is high.

A clear discussion of the use of genetic markers in paternity testing is given by Race and Sanger[9].

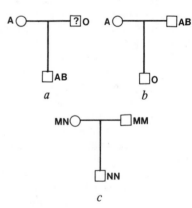

Fig. 7.5. Exclusion of paternity. *a,* ABO system. The child has antigen B, not present in mother or putative father. *b,* ABO system. The child has not inherited either of the putative father's A and B antigens (the mother must be hetero-zygous AO). *c,* MN system. The child is homozygous NN. One N has come from the mother, but the other N could not have come from the putative father, nor has the child received either of his M genes.

Exclusion of Paternity

It is always easier to exclude paternity than to establish it, and the exclusion is in general, accepted by the courts. Paternity can be excluded (assuming maternity is certain) by:

1. The child possessing a blood group antigen (or other genetic marker) not present in either parent.

2. The child not possessing an antigen for which the putative father is homozygous.

3. The child being homozygous for an antigen that the putative father does not possess.

Examples of these situations are given in *Fig. 7.5*.

The HLA system has proved the most polymorphic of all, excluding paternity in at least 75 per cent of cases. The blood groups are less effective individually, the ABO system excluding only 20 per cent of cases while the Rh and MNS systems will do so each in around 30 per cent.

The usual procedure is to use a combination of systems, including HLA and major blood groups, serum proteins and red cell enzymes already mentioned. This will allow exclusion of paternity in at least 95 per cent of cases.

Establishment of Paternity

This is much less certain than exclusion. By definition any alternative father is unavailable (otherwise he could be tested for exclusion). The approach used is to calculate the relative probability that the child has received a particular gene from the putative father, as compared with the chance that the gene may have come from an unknown member of the general population. If both father and child have the same rare antigen, this will clearly give heavy odds in favour of paternity, but in general, the evidence comes from the addition of numerous lesser odds. These may combine to give a total probability that leaves little doubt, but which never quite reaches 100 per cent and rarely carries the legal force that an exclusion of paternity gives.

Twins

Twin studies have played an important part in human genetics, but most of the available data are neither suitable nor relevant to genetic counselling. Only a few of the more important areas will be discussed here; some further reading is given at the end of this chapter. Twinning in relation to prenatal diagnosis is discussed in Chapter 6.

Determination of Zygosity

This may be simple, e.g. unlike sex twins must be dizygous. Triplets and other multiple pregnancies resulting from fertility drugs are likewise usually not monozygous. In a like sex twin pair, the most reliable clinical information comes from whether the twins consider themselves identical and are confused by others. This has been shown to correspond closely with detailed genotyping. Placentation is not a reliable guide. Wherever possible blood groups and HLA typing should be performed, which will allow exclusion of monozygosity in most cases. The approach to estimating probability of monozygosity is the same as for paternity testing.

Risks of Monozygous Twin Pairs

For a Mendelian disease, there should be complete concordance, i.e. both twins should either have or not have the disorder. There is often remarkable similarity in clinical features and age at onset.

For dominantly inherited disorders, an affected pair of monozygous twins with normal parents is compatible with a new mutation (unlike dizygous twins) and there is not an increased risk of the disease in subsequent children of the parents.

For non-Mendelian disorders, the risk to a co-twin will vary with the degree of genetic causation of the disease, being very high where genetic factors are predominant (as seen also in normal facial features and dermatoglyphics).

Risks of Dizygotic Twins

Since these are genetically no more alike than sibs, risks for Mendelian disorders are essentially the same as for sibs. For non-Mendelian conditions the shared intrauterine (and to some extent postnatal) environment gives a somewhat higher risk than that seen in sibs, but few accurate figures are available. In some instances concordance may be less than expected – thus in neural tube defects affected co-twins are exceptional and it is possible that such pregnancies are lost, a point of relevance when one twin is found to be abnormal in prenatal diagnosis.

Twinning in Families

Monozygous twins are rarely familial and have a rather constant incidence of around 4/1000 pregnancies. Dizygotic twinning, by contrast, shows marked geographical variation and frequently runs in families, particularly in the maternal line. Its frequency is around 6/1000 in European and White American populations, but it occurs in about 1 per cent of pregnancies in American Blacks, and up to 4 per cent of pregnancies in parts of Nigeria. The recurrence risk for dizygotic twins is about 1·7 per cent for Europeans.

Conjoined Twins

This phenomenon can be regarded as an extreme example of monozygotic twinning and is most unlikely to recur in a family. Ultrasound should now be able to give early warning of the problem.

References
1. Farrow M. G. and Juberg R. C. (1969) Genetics and laws prohibiting marriage in the United States. *JAMA* **209**, 534.
2. Schull W. J. (1958) Empirical risks in consanguineous marriages: sex ratio, malformation and viability. *Am. J. Genet.* **10**, 294–343.
3. Adams M. S. and Neel J. V. (1967) Children of incest. *Pediatrics* **40**, 55–62.
4. Carter C. O. (1967) Risk to offspring of incest. *Lancet* **1**, 436.

5. Seemanova E. (1971) A study of children of incestuous matings. *Hum. Genet.* **21,** 108–128.
6. Bundey S. (1970) The child of an incestuous union. In: Wolkind S. (ed.), *Medical Aspects of Adoption and Foster Care.* London, Heinemann, pp. 36–41.
7. McKusick V. A. (1978) *Medical Genetic Studies of the Amish.* Baltimore, Johns Hopkins University Press.
8. Williams E. M. and Harper P. S. (1977) Genetic study of Welsh gypsies. *J. Med. Genet.* **14,** 172–176.
9. Race R. R. and Sanger R. (1975) *Blood Groups in Man.* 6th ed. Oxford, Blackwell.

Further Reading
Bulmer M. G. (1970) *The Biology of Twinning in Man.* Oxford, Clarendon Press.
Emery A. E. H. (1976) *Methodology in Medical Genetics.* London, Churchill Livingstone.
Shields J. (1962) *Monozygotic Twins Brought up Apart and Brought up Together.* London, Oxford University Press.

CHAPTER EIGHT

The Genetic Counselling Clinic

The primary aim of this book has been to encourage clinicians to regard genetic counselling as an integral part of the management of patients and their families, and to dispel the view that any genetic problem must of necessity be referred to a specialist clinic. Nevertheless, the organizational aspects of genetic counselling require careful consideration, whoever is doing it, and the following notes are intended to cover some of the practical aspects which need close attention if an efficient and successful service is to be provided for patients.

General Aspects

1. *Time*

Adequate time is essential if genetic counselling is to be at all worthwhile, and it may be argued that the main advantage of a patient being seen in a specialist genetic clinic is the greater amount of time that a medical geneticist is likely to be able to devote to the problem, than can most busy clinicians. All too often patients complain not that their doctor advised them incorrectly, but that he was too busy to answer their questions adequately or even to appreciate that the problem existed.

Clearly the first duty of a doctor interested in his patients' genetic problems is to ensure that this time is provided. The author finds one hour to be the usual time required to take full pedigree details, undertake examination of a patient, and discuss the genetic risks. A follow-up visit is frequently required to interpret the results of investigations or records that have been obtained on relatives, and half an hour is usually allowed for this. Investigation of an extended family may take considerably longer and it is wise to attempt this in stages. The arrival of a complete kindred of upwards of a dozen people can create consternation in a clinic, while the conflicting views of several branches of a family are also best dealt with separately!

2. *Setting*

The necessity of adequate time usually means that a specific session is best set aside for genetic counselling, whether this be in a family doctor's office or surgery, or in a hospital clinician's outpatient department. Whatever the precise location, several needs must be borne in mind. *Quiet and freedom from disturbance* are essential. The design of many hospital outpatient departments makes this almost impossible, while the rumpus associated with most childrens' clinics is also a distraction. A room without a telephone is an advantage, and the coming and going of well-meaning nurses must be discouraged. The author has found it necessary to place a sign 'Genetic counselling, do not disturb' on the door.

The number of people present must be small if patients are not to be inhibited in discussing personal details, usually not more than one medical colleague and a social worker. A single student can perhaps be added, but pressure to accommodate large student or postgraduate groups should be resisted. One-way screens are sometimes advocated to avoid this problem, but the author dislikes them.

If the clinic is held in a paediatric setting, there must be facilities for examining adults also; the unexpected emergence of a large undressed adult in the midst of a paediatric clinic may cause anxiety.

3. Equipment
Very little is needed. It is a pleasure in these days of high cost technology and centralization to be able to provide a high class service to people in a relatively remote area without the need for cumbersome equipment or excessive cost to the community (or to the patient). A full set of examination equipment is essential, for many patients sent for counselling will prove really to need diagnosis. Facilities for blood taking and for x-rays (especially skelatal) are helpful; samples for most laboratory tests, including cytogenetic studies, can be taken at a distance if necessary, and brought back to the central laboratory for analysis.

4. Pedigrees and Records
The number of families seen increases with a remarkable rapidity, and unless a clear and simple system is decided on from the outset, the clinician will soon find himself unable to find relevant information. The keeping of systematic records is also the foundation for much of the research on inherited disorders, and should allow for follow-up and long-term preventive measures where appropriate.

A clear and detailed pedigree is the foundation of good genetic counselling and a simple lined sheet is useful to keep it neat and orderly. The temptation to construct a rough pedigree for later improvement should be resisted — time and energy are rarely enough for this to actually happen! With practice a clear pedigree can be produced quite quickly, using the method and symbols described in Chapter 1. Relevant pieces of information can be placed at the bottom, using letters to identify the particular individuals. *Fig.* 1.2, p. 7 shows typical pedigrees on the author's pedigree chart.

Other medical details will also need recording and in the author's clinic the policy has always been to write these in the regular hospital case-record, where a copy of all correspondence is also placed. A copy of such notes and letters, along with the pedigree, is kept in the Medical Genetics Department, where it is immediately available for consultation, in contrast to the main hospital case-record which may be in use elsewhere or missing.

An easily workable index system is vital, especially in regions like Wales where many unrelated people share the same few surnames. It can be embarrassing to discover that the Mrs Davies that one thought had a child with Duchenne dystrophy is, in fact, at risk for Huntington's chorea! Computerized registers may have a place in a large specialist unit, but for most clinicians a simple card index will suffice. The author's policy is for each *kindred* to be allotted a unique serial number and for all members of it to share this number. Each member seen (or on whom relevant details exist) has a separate index card giving name, address, date of birth, etc., but shares the same family number and a single folder in which details on the family are kept. Cards are filed alphabetically and a separate diagnosis index is kept.

This system, borrowed from that used at the Moore Clinic, Baltimore, is probably suitable for up to 10 000 family records; it is not perfect, but is flexible and easy to maintain.

The Genetic Advisory Service

This chapter has so far concentrated on the provision of genetic counselling by clinicians who are not specialists in medical genetics. There will always be patients who require a specialist referral, however, and at present the awareness of genetic problems and consequent need for genetic counselling is growing faster than the ability of general clinicians to provide it. Many countries, including Britain, have evolved a system of regional genetic advisory centres to provide a specialist service, and since resources are limited and potential demand very large it is important to consider how these are best utilized by doctors and other referring personnel.

In Britain, there is now a genetic advisory centre in most hospital administrative regions, usually based in the medical teaching centre of the region concerned, and commonly staffed by or closely associated with an academic medical genetics unit. There is often a close link with cytogenetic and other laboratory services. Hospital regions commonly serve a population of 2–6 million people, and vary in their area. The author's own service covers Wales, with a population of 3 million and a maximum distance of 200 miles from the teaching centre. Here, as in some other regions, a service of regular 'satellite clinics' has been set up to serve more distant parts of the region, which are run in cooperation with local clinicians and are serviced from the main unit in the medical teaching centre. In addition to this regional service, a number of specialist clinics have been set up with interested clinicians to deal with particular problems, for example congenital deafness, blindness and plastic surgery disorders.

The source of referrals to the author's clinics is almost equally divided between family doctors and hospital clinicians, with smaller numbers from community health doctors and social workers. Self-referrals are common, but are channelled through family doctors. The breakdown by diagnosis of a personal series of 1000 referrals is shown in *Table* 8.1. Although the prominence of neurological disorders reflects the author's own interests, there is no doubt that this group ranks very high among the major problems in genetic counselling.

Table 8.1. Referrals to Genetic Counselling Clinic (1000 consecutive referrals; pre-amniocentesis counselling and research visits excluded)

		%
Congenital malformations	Neural tube defects	8·5
	Chromosome anomalies	5·1
	Other malformations	4·1
Inherited neurological disorders	Huntington's chorea	9·5
	Muscular dystrophies	12·4
	Mental retardation (non-specific)	2·5
	Others	8·7
Skeletal disorders		12·7
Inherited metabolic disorders		13·3
Inherited disorders of other systems		15·7
Obstetric-gynaecological problems (excluding prenatal diagnosis)		6·4
Consanguinity		1·1

The genetic advisory service in the UK has evolved historically within the framework of the National Health Service and thus differs in many ways from the pattern seen in much of continental Europe and the USA. It may well prove to be one of the major and lasting achievements of the British National Health Service that the development of medical genetics has been able to take place relatively painlessly inside this service, and that the provision of a sound, even though restricted service has been possible without the necessity for charging of fees to patients or relatives. This applies equally to the provision of cytogenetic and prenatal diagnostic services. Whether the existing structure of services will prove adequate to cope with the steady increase in demand remains to be seen, and will depend largely on to what extent clinicians are prepared and able to undertake genetic counselling for families under their own care.

Non-medical Staff and Genetic Counselling

Twenty years ago most genetic counselling was undertaken by non-medically trained geneticists for the simple reason that very few physicians had any knowledge of or interest in genetics. The situation now is entirely different, and the great majority of genetic counselling is done by medically trained staff with some form of training (often it has to be said inadequate!) in genetics. The rapid development of such areas as prenatal diagnosis, screening and early therapy, together with the delineation of numerous clinically recognizable syndromes, has made it difficult for the non-medical geneticist to remain in the front line of clinical genetics, even though most of the underlying biochemical and cytogenetic research responsible for these advances has been made by non-medical scientists.

The author believes strongly that genetic counselling should preferably be undertaken by people who are medically trained, largely for the reason that it is quite impossible to separate the actual counselling from the associated aspects of clinical diagnosis. On numerous occasions, what is referred as an apparently straightforward problem of risk estimation and counselling produces a completely unexpected diagnostic problem, that a non-medical person would not only not be able to solve, but might well fail to recognize. For this reason the training of large numbers of non-medical 'genetic counsellors' does not seem to be the logical answer to increasing demand, although this approach has been attempted in some American centres.

To avoid incurring too much wrath from his many non-medical friends and colleagues, the author would straight away recognize that many geneticists without medical training continue to provide first rate genetic counselling, learning to recognize their diagnostic limitation and acquiring through experience considerable clinical skills. Conversely, there are still too many medically qualified people in the field whose knowledge of basic genetics is at best minimal. Nevertheless, in planning for the future, the author is in no doubt that training in both medicine and genetics is desirable for those intending to devote all or much of their time to genetic counselling. It may be argued that to train such individuals is expensive; this is true, but it is preferable to have a relatively small number of well-trained people and for them to be used selectively. This view returns to the underlying theme of this book — that most genetic counselling is and will continue to be done by regular clinicians as a part of the overall management of patients under their care, while the medical geneticist is principally involved in those families where the situation is less simple, and in educating his clinical colleagues.

In a number of centres, the preliminary process of drawing up a pedigree and eliciting family information is done by an auxiliary worker before the family is seen by the medical geneticist. It can certainly be argued that this saves valuable medical time, but the author does not personally favour it. Taking the family details gives a valuable opportunity to 'break the ice' and form a relationship with a family being seen for the first time; a lot can be learned about their fears and worries, their general attitude to the disorder in the family, how well they are likely to understand risk figures, and whether there are disagreements and tensions within the family. On several occasions it has become quite clear during the process that someone coming primarily for counselling is affected by the disorder; Huntington's chorea is an example of such a condition, where a period of quiet observation during history-taking may give much more information than a formal examination.

In addition to the non-medical geneticist, other non-medical staff have valuable roles to play in the genetic counselling clinic. An experienced and sensitive social worker will often be able to detect problems that the family have not spoken about, and ensure that they have actually understood what the person giving genetic counselling thinks they have – the two often prove surprisingly different! In many instances, practical support may need to be arranged; this may be as valuable as the genetic counselling itself.

The author has also been fortunate in having the services of an experienced nurse acting as field worker, whose help is invaluable in contacting relatives at home, taking samples from relatives, and obtaining additional information left incomplete at the time of a clinic visit. It is difficult to provide more than a very limited genetic counselling service without the availability of such non-medical staff.

The Back-up to Genetic Counselling

Genetic counselling does not happen in a vacuum. The topics of carrier detection and prenatal diagnosis have already been discussed, but there are a number of other practical aspects that arise in connection with genetic counselling and which are dealt with here.

Contraception

Ready access to a family planning clinic is essential for any clinician involved in genetic counselling, and it is always wise to enquire tactfully about contraception at an early stage, particularly if the results of investigations are going to take some weeks or months before definitive counselling can be given. It is surprising how often couples aware of the genetic risk and not intending to have children nevertheless take no active measures to prevent pregnancy. The author has more than once had the unhappy experience of seeing a couple on follow-up visit, to give a high risk of a serious disorder, only to find that the wife has become pregnant in the meantime.

Sterilization

This is often preferable to long-term contraception where a couple has made a definite decision not to have further children. This may apply even to young people. Before sterilization is undertaken, however, careful consideration must be given to the following points:

1. What is the precise genetic risk to offspring? It is not uncommon for sterilization to be requested 'on genetic grounds' when the risks of trans-

mitting a disorder are negligible, e.g. sibs of a patient with an autosomal recessive disorder.

2. Is there an alternative such as carrier detection or prenatal diagnosis, that could reduce or avoid the risk?

3. Is it likely that advances in knowledge will change the situation in the next few years?

4. Do the couple really agree that sterilization is the best course and which partner should undergo it?

In general it is logical to sterilize the affected or at-risk individual in the case of a dominant disease; for autosomal recessive disorders there is no genetic preference; many couples choose vasectomy on grounds of simplicity and lesser risk. In some instances the unaffected member of a couple insists on being sterilized; the motivation in such circumstances can be complex. In the case of a fatal disorder the possibility that the healthy spouse may remarry and wish to have children must be faced.

Sterilization of the mentally handicapped is a difficult and emotive issue. Genetic risks to offspring are often confused with the more general questions concerning whether a child could be satisfactorily reared by the parents. Despite the recent arguments over the rights of the handicapped to reproduce, sterilization seems a perfectly reasonable course if the retardation is more than mild, the genetic risks high and the risk of pregnancy considerable. The right of a child to be born where possible into a healthy family does not seem to have received sufficient attention in discussion of this issue.

Artificial Insemination by Donor (AID)

AID has a limited but definite role in relation to genetic counselling. Its use is currently limited by social rather than by technical factors, and it is important for clinicians to be aware of its potential and limitations even though its widespread use seems unlikely in the near future.

Techniques of artificial insemination were originally developed for use in animal husbandry and are now in routine use for a variety of species. Experience in this field has clearly shown that donor semen can be stored in liquid nitrogen without significant loss of viability, and without significant fetal loss or increased risk of abnormality in the subsequent offspring. Artificial insemination has in fact played a valuable eugenic role in making available semen from high quality pedigree stock to farmers in the most remote areas.

The use of AID in man has so far been mainly in cases of male infertility; this experience has confirmed that obtained from animals in that successful pregnancy can regularly be obtained (though up to 3 inseminations are commonly required) and there is no obvious increase in malformations or abortions. The use of the technique in relation to inherited disease is essentially identical. A time close to ovulation is chosen. The semen is introduced by a fine pipette into the cervix (a painless procedure) and the patient lies flat for at least one hour by which time it is hoped that it will have achieved fertilization.

The main *potential* genetic indications for AID are as follows:

1. Autosomal dominant disorders where the male is affected or at risk of becoming so (e.g. Huntington's chorea).

2. Rare autosomal recessive disorders, in particular where prenatal diagnosis is not feasible or termination of pregnancy not acceptable to the couple. Here a gene must be contributed by each parent and an unrelated donor is most unlikely to carry the gene.

3. Polygenic disorders where a concentration of affected individuals exists solely on the male side. Here there is much less certainty of avoiding recurrence, especially if an affected child has already been born to the couple, since the abnormal genetic contribution is rarely confined to the one side.

In choosing donors, it must be ensured that they are anonymous, healthy, reasonably intelligent, without any family history of genetic disorders, and unrelated to the recipient. In practice, medical students are usually chosen — more for reasons of convenience than because they best fulfil the above criteria!

The drawbacks of AID are, from the medical and technical viewpoint very small. There are, however, two major non-medical limitations which have so far limited its use.

1. The legal situation. This remains confused, both in the UK and in the USA. In practice, almost all couples register the birth as their own child, and this is clearly the desirable course. In strict legal terms this may be incorrect, but this has never been tested and it is clearly a situation where the law has not yet caught up with a situation that did not exist when laws were framed.

2. Many couples find AID unacceptable, even when the genetic indications would appear suitable. This may be because they find the idea distasteful, or because one parent is being excluded from the reproductive process, in contrast to adoption, where both parents share in the bringing up of a child that is not biologically their own, and where the process is generally openly acknowledged. As with many aspects of genetic counselling, AID may throw added strain on a marriage that is already in difficulties, and it is certainly not a procedure to undertake without ensuring that its consequences have been fully understood and accepted by both members of the couple.

Because human AID is a relatively recent development, there is still little information on its long-term consequences. Confidentiality is a particular problem. The development of registers and data banks makes this information hard to conceal if it is recorded in medical notes, but if it is not, the individual may at some future date be regarded as being at risk for the very genetic disorder which AID was used to avoid. Likewise, it is difficult to know whether parents should be advised to tell the child at some stage of his true origin, or if so, at what stage. Until some information on these problems is available, it seems unwise to consider the large-scale use of AID. The most important factor of all, but also the least predictable, is the climate of public opinion. It is possible that this may change quite rapidly regarding AID, as it has regarding abortion. Responsible use of the procedure is likely to help considerably in its general acceptance.

Embryo Transfer

It is now technically feasible (though extremely difficult) to remove unfertilized ova after ovulation, to perform *in vitro* fertilization and then to reimplant the fertilized ovum into the uterus. So far in man this has been done using both sperm and ovum from an infertile couple, but there is no technical reason why ova from an unrelated female donor cannot be used.

Although the genetic and legal problems are no greater than those of AID, it is likely that public acceptance will be even more reluctant. Nevertheless the author has already had serious enquiries about using the technique from mildly affected women with variable dominantly inherited disorders. X-linked recessive disorders would also be a potential field for its application, particularly where prenatal diagnostic tests do not exist.

Adoption

The question of adoption in relation to genetic counselling arises in two main situations:

1. Adoption is being considered as one of the options open to a couple at risk of transmitting a genetic disorder.

2. A child being placed for adoption has a family history of a genetic disorder and the adoption agency wishes to know how great the risk is before finalizing the placement.

Until recently, it was possible to recommend adoption as a possible course of action for couples not wishing to take the risk of having a natural child with a genetic disorder. With increasing use of abortion for social indications and a trend towards single mothers retaining their children, the number of available children has decreased sharply, and couples with a family history of genetic disease will thus find themselves competing with many healthy, but infertile couples for a small number of children.

In these circumstances, couples are often discouraged even from considering adoption, but I feel strongly that this course is wrong and that if a couple want to adopt, they should attempt to do so. They should realize, however, that considerable determination is needed, since a large amount of 'red tape' and bureaucratic inertia may be encountered that will discourage the faint hearted. The following advice may help:

Apply early since a long wait may be inevitable.

If one agency states that their list is closed try others, in another region if necessary – a serious lack of communication between agencies and areas exists.

Be prepared to be inspected, questioned and to fill out a large number of forms.

If barriers of religion are raised, work through a local authority or other non-denominational agency.

Be persistent (without being aggressive) if delays occur.

Consider the adoption of an older child, or one with some other reason that has made adoption difficult.

Because many couples feel helpless in how to start adopting some further information is included in the appendix (p. 270).

One group of people who may have particular difficulty in adopting are those where one partner is at high risk of actually developing a serious genetic disorder, such as Huntington's chorea. Here a decision must be made in each case based on a careful evaluation of the size of the risk, the chance that the disease will develop while the child is being brought up and the nature of the disorder. For a condition with such serious consequences as Huntington's chorea, few adoption agencies will feel able to accept a couple at high risk.

Adoption and the Child at Risk
Advice is commonly sought from adoption agencies when a child to be placed for adoption has a family history of a serious disorder. Sadly this advice is rarely sought *before* the birth of the child, with the result that unnecessary delay may occur, with resulting uncertainty and harm to the infant, natural mother and adoptive parents alike. The estimation of risks is no different from that in other genetic counselling situations, though unavailability (or uncertainty) of the father may cause difficulty. A more difficult problem is where the child results from an incestuous mating (*see* Chapter 7) where the risks are for a variety of recessively inherited disorders, not all of which are detectable in infancy. In this situation, and in such disorders as Duchenne muscular dystrophy, it may be wise to defer placement for a few months until the major part of the risk can be excluded.

Where a high risk of a late onset disorder does exist, many infants are excluded from adoption. This seems unfortunate, since from the child's viewpoint a family will certainly be likely to deal with problems that arise better than an institution will; it is also often overlooked that there are many highly motivated couples who are prepared to adopt or foster long-term children with even very severe disabilities provided that they are fully in the picture as to what they are taking on; very few children should be considered 'unsuitable for adoption'.

Genetic Registers
The keeping of accurate and complete records is an essential, though often neglected, part of all branches of clinical medicine, but the long term and

preventive nature of medical genetics makes this a specially important aspect. Much of the information given in genetic counselling may only be fully used many years later: the sister of a boy with Duchenne muscular dystrophy or the child of a patient with polyposis coli may have been too young to be given any information at the time of the initial family study; unless careful records are kept, investigations may have to be repeated. Likewise it is of great help to know that a person with vague neurological symptoms and a family history of possible Huntington's chorea is in fact a member of a kindred where the diagnosis has been fully established.

Table 8.2. Disorders worth considering for a preventive genetic register

X-linked recessive
        Duchenne muscular dystrophy
        Becker muscular dystrophy
        Haemophilia (A and B)
        Other serious rare X-linked disorders

Autosomal dominant
        Polyposis coli (and other inherited neoplastic syndromes)
        Polycystic kidney disease
        Huntington's chorea
        Retinitis pigmentosa (also X-linked form)
        Myotonic dystrophy
        Marfan syndrome

Chromosomal
        Translocation Down's syndrome (and related translocations)

A genetic register is something more than an accurate records system. The term 'register' implies that the approach is systematic and at least aiming at completeness, and that the information is actively maintained and updated. Genetic registers may be of several types and can vary in complexity from a simple card index to a complex computerized system.

a. Disease specific register. This is the type likely to be of greatest interest to the practising clinician with a special interest in a particular group of inherited disorders. Here the genetic aspects are only part of the objective, and a register may be of considerable help in overall management and in research, as well as in genetic counselling. Regional registers for such conditions as haemophilia, polyposis coli and cystic fibrosis are examples.

b. Preventive registers. Here the specific aim is to allow genetic counselling and other preventive measures to be applied in inherited disorders where there may be numerous family members at risk who might be unaware of the problem. The most suitable disorders for such a register (*Table* 8.2) are the late onset dominant disorders such as polycystic kidney disease and Huntington's chorea, or X-linked disorders such as

Duchenne and Becker muscular dystrophy. Here an accurate knowledge of affected and at risk individuals in a region is likely to be of considerable help in ensuring that genetic counselling is provided early rather than when an affected or potentially affected child has already been born. By contrast, autosomal recessive disorders, the common polygenic conditions and chromosomal abnormalities (apart from translocations) are not suitable for this type of register since the risks are either low or are confined to the immediate family which is likely to be aware of them already.

Other types of register may be used to monitor the effects of amniocentesis or other procedures, but these are mainly of use to the specialist medical genetics unit. A full discussion can be found in a recent report of a Working Party of the Clinical Genetics Society. Before the reader becomes too enthusiastic about the subject, however, some problems should be considered:

1. How can one keep the register specific and limited? It is all too easy for its scope to expand until it is out of control (one 'high-risk children' register known to the author was found to include more than half the children in the area!). It is better to confine oneself to a small number of well-defined conditions and deal with them thoroughly.

2. How can one maintain the quality of the information? An inaccurate or out-of-date register is worse than useless. Accepting data at face value from outside sources is dangerous, and in general, the only person likely to have sufficient sustained enthusiasm to check the information thoroughly is the person actually maintaining the register. It must also be recognized that updating a register entails a lot of work and that the expense is also not negligible.

3. Confidentiality. This may not be much of a problem for a socially acceptable disorder like haemophilia, but in a disease such as Huntington's chorea it is of the utmost significance. It is essential that *no* information is given out without the permission of the individuals concerned, that the register is kept securely, and that no identifying details are put on any computerized system. The author's experience, gained chiefly from a register of muscular dystrophies and Huntington's chorea, is that most individuals are extremely helpful provided that they can have a personal relationship with those running the register. If it is under bureaucratic control or any information is divulged without permission, this cooperation would almost certainly be lost.

Further Reading (*see also* Chapter 1)

Emery A. E. H., Brough C., Crawfurd M. et al. (1978) A report on Genetic Registers. *J Med. Genet.* **15**, 435–442.

Lubs H. A. and De La Cruz F. (ed.) (1977) *Genetic Counseling.* New York, Raven Press.

Milunsky A. and Annas G. J. (ed.) (1976) *Genetics and The Law.* New York, Plenum.

Wolkind E. S. (ed.) (1979) *Medical Aspects of Adoption and Foster Care.* London, Heinemann.

II. Specific Organ Systems

CHAPTER NINE

Neuromuscular Disease

Muscular Dystrophies

Too often patients are referred for genetic counselling or even worse, for prenatal procedures, with a label of 'muscular dystrophy' and no indication as to the type of dystrophy concerned. Most laymen (and some doctors!) have the impression that all muscular dystrophy affects boys, but is carried by girls. The first task in genetic counselling is thus clearly to establish the precise diagnosis beyond all reasonable doubt. *Table* 9.1 lists the major categories of muscular dystrophy and their inheritance.

Table 9.1. The progressive muscular dystrophies

Duchenne dystrophy Becker dystrophy Emery–Dreifuss type	X-linked recessive
Early onset 'Duchenne-like' girdle dystrophy Limb girdle dystrophy (Erb)	Autosomal recessive
Facioscapulohumeral Distal Oculopharyngeal	Autosomal dominant
Myotonic dystrophy	Autosomal dominant

Duchenne Muscular Dystrophy

Duchenne muscular dystrophy is one of the major problems in genetic counselling, particularly for paediatricians and neurologists. Its X-linked recessive mode of inheritance means that numerous female relations may be at risk of being carriers, even with a single case in the family; it is essential that they are advised accurately and that both genetic and bio-chemical information is used correctly in determining carrier status. At present this is often not the case, and the resulting misinformation may lead to disastrous results for the family concerned.

The only other established preventive measure, apart from carrier detection, is fetal sex determination for pregnancies of definite or high-risk carriers; prenatal diagnosis from levels of creatine kinase in fetal blood has been advocated but there is no clear evidence yet of its reliability. In testing infants at risk, creatine kinase in cord blood is extremely variable and is best avoided. Likewise, there is dispute as to whether neonatal screening for the disease (to prevent subsequent affected children being bórn before the first in a family has been recognized) is desirable. All of this adds to the importance of accurate genetic counselling and carrier detection.

Carrier detection. The general problems of calculating risks for a lethal X-linked disorder have already been discussed (Chapters 2 and 5). A woman with two affected sons or with one affected son and another affected close male relative is clearly an *obligatory* carrier, with a 50 per cent risk of further sons being affected and of daughters being carriers.

Prior risks for various degrees of relationship are shown in *Fig.* 9.1; in general each generation removed from the affected person halves the prior

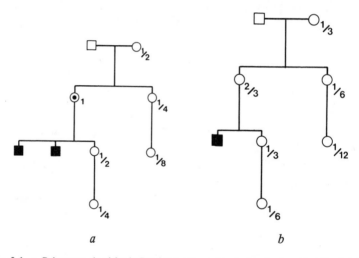

a   *b*

Fig. 9.1. *a,* Prior genetic risks in Duchenne muscular dystrophy (*see* text for details). *b,* Prior genetic risks in an isolated case of Duchenne myscular dystrophy (*see* text for details).

risk. Isolated cases are a special problem. Although there has been argument over the proportion of these which represent new mutations, the observed data suggest that the risk for the mother of a new case being a carrier is 2/3, and that the risk of the grandmother also being a carrier is 1/3 (*Fig.* 9.1*b*).

The prior risk should not be used alone in counselling but should be combined with other (conditional) genetic information and with information from carrier testing. In practice this means use of serum creatine kinase; other methods give little extra information. A few women show overt muscle weakness but are usually those where carrier testing also gives clear-cut results. Careful muscle testing may show a lesser degree of weakness in asymptomatic carriers and is always worth performing.

Serum creatine kinase (CK). Few tests have been so misused as this, and if the clinician is not prepared to take considerable trouble over taking samples and interpreting results, and does not have access to a reliable laboratory with a properly defined normal range, it is better that the test is not done at all.

Details of handling of samples for CK analysis are given elsewhere[1], but they should be taken under conditions of normal activity, and transported promptly to the laboratory. Factors such as age, pregnancy, therapy and unrelated diseases must be taken into account, and the mean of three results used to calculate risks.

The sensitivity of serum creatine kinase in detecting the carrier state of Duchenne muscular dystrophy is considerably increased by using odds or

Table 9.2. Likelihood of being a carrier for different levels of serum creatine kinase (CK) (Based on data of Sibert et al., 1979)

CK (iu/l)	Likelihood ratio	Probability	CK	Likelihood ratio	Probability
<40	0·12	0·11	120–	12·79	0·93
40–	0·12	0·11	130–	25·12	0·96
50–	0·16	0·14	140–	49·02	0·98
60–	0·27	0·22	150–	94·34	0·99
70–	0·46	0·32	160–	180·9	0·995
80–	0·86	0·46	170–	342·5	0·997
90–	1·67	0·63	180–	641·0	0·998
100–	3·28	0·77	190+	>1000	>0·999
110–	6·49	0·87			

N.B. These figures are based on an upper limit (95 per cent) of normal for adult females of 100 iu/l and cannot be applied unmodified to other methods of analysis. Anyone utilizing creatine kinase levels in genetic counselling should ensure that their laboratory range has been accurately standardised and if possible expressed in terms of odds as above. These odds should only be used in conjunction with the genetic risks (*see* text).

likelihood ratios for specific values of CK rather than considering results as 'normal' or 'abnormal' (*Table* 9.2). This is particularly critical where the result is within the 'normal' range as occurs in one-third of cases – it can be seen that while a 'low normal' value will strongly favour normality, a 'high normal' result may actually favour the carrier state.

It can also be seen that there is a neutral point (likelihood ratio 1), where the results neither increase nor decrease the chances of being a carrier.

Finally, it must be stressed that these odds are *not* the risk of a woman being a carrier. They must be interpreted in the light of the prior genetic risk and any other available information if gross errors are to be avoided. Wherever possible all potential carriers in a family should be tested together, since the results on one member may significantly influence the risk for others.

The age at which potential carriers should be tested is debatable. In general the author is reluctant to test young girls because of lack of obligatory carriers in this age group and of knowledge regarding their normal range of CK. Recent evidence suggests that the serum CK of normal girls around the menarche is higher than that of adults, so that odds based on slightly raised levels should be regarded as provisional in this group [2]. During pregnancy CK levels are markedly reduced, and carrier testing in pregnancy is likely to lead to serious errors.

If the above comments seem to make an easy test appear difficult, no apologies are offered. The use and interpretation of CK and the calculation of risks in carrier detection of Duchenne dystrophy can on occasion be extremely difficult and always requires great care. It is particularly important that the risks of potential carriers are worked out *before* such procedures as fetal sexing (and possibly prenatal diagnosis using fetal blood in future) are considered.

Population Screening for Duchenne Muscular Dystrophy. The exceptionally high levels of serum CK seen in presymptomatic cases of Duchenne dystrophy leave no doubt that affected males (not carriers) can be detected soon after birth. Cord blood values are too variable for this, but it has been suggested that population screening of males could be undertaken using the newborn samples collected on filter paper for phenylketonuria testing [3]. Although this is almost certainly feasible there is serious doubt whether this approach is justified at present, for a number of reasons. First, there is no effective treatment; thus the justification would be to prevent the birth of future cases in the families of presymptomatic affected infants. Whether the distress likely to be caused in these families (and the families who prove to be 'false-positives') is outweighed by the resulting benefits is questionable [4]. Secondly, since one-third of cases are thought to be new mutants (with no risk to other family members), while half of the remaining two-thirds born to carrier mothers are also isolated cases, it would seem unlikely that population screening would reduce the incidence of the disease by more than one-third.

The author's opinion is that efforts should at present be concentrated on ensuring that the families of known cases are fully and accurately tested, and that comprehensive registers of known and probable carriers are kept in all regions. It seems premature to embark on screening until the more limited but essential task of carrier detection in known families has been achieved.

Becker (late onset X-linked) Dystrophy

Distinction from Duchenne dystrophy is important in giving an accurate prognosis, though the inheritance and genetic risks are essentially similar. The proportion of carriers showing elevated CK levels is lower than in Duchenne dystrophy (around 50 per cent)[5]. Reproduction of affected males is common; *all* daughters will be carriers, regardless of CK level, while all sons will be healthy. In isolated cases or those confined to sibs the autosomal recessive limb-girdle dystrophy must be distinguished (*see below*).

Other Progressive Muscle Dystrophies (*see Table 9.1*)

Facioscapulohumeral dystrophy is frequently mild and individuals at risk must be carefully examined before being accepted as normal. A young adult who is *entirely* normal on examination is unlikely to develop or transmit the disorder. CK is of little help in early detection; levels may be normal in mild or presymptomatic cases.

Autosomal recessive limb girdle dystrophy in a male may be difficult to distinguish from Becker dystrophy — risks will be quite different and fetal sexing inappropriate. Mild cases in women can be confused with the rare 'manifesting carriers' of Duchenne dystrophy. In both sexes confusion with benign spinal muscular atrophy is possible, but the inheritance is the same.

Table 9.3. Congenital myopathies

	Inheritance
Nemaline myopathy	Autosomal dominant
Myotubular (centronuclear) myopathy)	Autosomal recessive
Central core disease	Autosomal dominant
Congenital fibre type disproportion	Uncertain
Congenital myotonic dystrophy	Autosomal dominant

Congenital Myopathies (*Table 9.3*)

Unless the pattern of inheritance within a particular family is clear cut, genetic counselling for this heterogeneous group should not be undertaken without an accurate muscle biopsy diagnosis from a competent centre. Variation in severity within families may be marked.

Myotonic Dystrophy

This autosomal dominant disorder, for long a special interest of the author, ranks second only to Duchenne dystrophy as a major counselling problem in inherited muscle disease. Its extreme clinical variability adds special difficulty.

Definitely affected people have a 50 per cent risk for affected offspring. Affected women, even if mildly affected, have a considerable risk (*Table* 9.4) that an affected child will have the severe childhood form of the disease [6], which may result in neonatal death, severe respiratory problems after birth and severe physical and mental handicap in survivors; the risk is especially high where a women has already had such an affected child. The risk of this form in the offspring of affected males is small. Although clinical severity of disease does show some correlation within families, variation within a family is so great that a mildly affected individual has no guarantee that the disease will remain so in subsequent generations.

Table 9.4. Risks for offspring of women with myotonic dystrophy (from Harper 1979)

	%
Normal	50·0
Neonatal deaths and stillbirths	12·0
Severely affected — surviving	9·0
Later affected	29·0

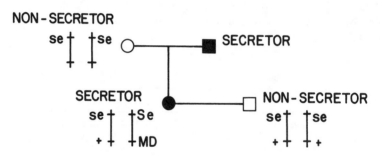

Fig. 9.2. Risk prediction in myotonic dystrophy using the linked secretor locus. (Family studied by courtesy of Professor C. O. Carter.) From Harper, (1979). Secretor offspring would be expected to be affected.

Genetic advice to family members at risk must be preceded by thorough examination and by electromyography and slit-lamp examination for lens opacities. My own study found 15 per cent of asymptomatic first-degree relatives to show clinical abnormalities while the other investigations detected another 5 per cent of gene carriers [7]. Where scanty lens opacities are the only abnormality, they should be counted since normal individuals may have small numbers. However thoroughly individuals are studied it is likely that a small proportion appearing normal will later develop abnormalities. Those found to be normal in childhood should be re-assessed prior to having a family. No reliable biochemical predictive test has yet been found; CK is often normal in early stages, though a raised value should give rise to suspicion.

Genetic linkage between the myotonic dystrophy and secretor loci allows prediction of whether an individual will develop the disorder in a proportion (around 1/5) of families, but has a built-in error of at least 10 per cent due to crossing-over between the loci. The test can be done simply on saliva. It can also be used in prenatal prediction from amniotic fluid, though the same drawbacks apply[7]. Those families that can be helped by amniocentesis can be identified by prior saliva testing as shown in *Fig.* 9.2 (*see also* Chapter 6).

Myotonic dystrophy is frequently characterized by inertia and apathy, and the gene is transmitted largely by individuals who do not consider themselves to be abnormal. New mutations are extremely rare. An active approach to testing and advising family members is thus essential if any impact is to be made; this is particularly justified in the case of mildly affected women whose offspring are at risk of the severe congenital form of the disease.

Table 9.5. The myotonic syndromes

	Inheritance
Myotonic dystrophy	Autosomal dominant
Myotonia congenita	
a. Thomsen's disease	Autosomal dominant
b. Recessive type	Autosomal recessive
c. With painful cramps	Autosomal dominant
Paramyotonia congenita	Autosomal dominant
Periodic paralysis	
a. Hypokalaemic	Autosomal dominant
b. Normo/hyperkalaemic (adynamia episodica)	Autosomal dominant
Chondrodystrophic myotonia	Autosomal recessive
(Schwartz–Jampel syndrome)	
Acquired myotonia	
a. Drug induced	–
b. Associated with malignancy	

Other Myotonic Syndromes (*Table* 9.5)

All are rare in comparison with myotonic dystrophy which must be carefully excluded. *Myotonia congenita* (Thomsen's disease) is heterogeneous and at least half the cases are recessively inherited, despite the prominence of some large dominantly inherited families. The two types show clinical as well as genetic differences. Since new mutations for this benign condition are likely to be rare, it is wise to give a 1 in 4 risk for further children born to healthy parents of an isolated case. Correspondingly the risk of such an isolated case transmitting the condition is small.

Spinal Muscular Atrophies

This heterogeneous group of anterior horn cell disorders requires careful distinction on clinical, electromyographic and histological grounds from primary myopathies. The great majority of all types follow autosomal recessive inheritance, so that sporadic cases should be counselled as such even if it is difficult to assign them to a particular type. Prenatal diagnosis is not feasible at present.

Type I

Severe infantile spinal muscular atrophy (Werdnig–Hoffmann disease) (autosomal recessive). Onset is at or shortly after birth, with death invariably before 2 years and usually before 18 months. Severity in other affected sibs is closely correlated[8], so that couples taking the 1 in 4 risk of recurrence can be reassured that the risk of a severely handicapped *surviving* child is minimal and that a sib apparently healthy at 6 months old will almost certainly remain normal.

Type II

Chronic childhood spinal muscular atrophy. This group includes those cases with childhood onset, but survival beyond two years. The majority are severely handicapped during childhood. Occasional X-linked families have been reported, but are too rare compared with autosomal recessive cases to affect counselling for isolated male cases. Variability between sibs is greater than for the infantile type, but an apparently healthy sib will have passed through 90 per cent of its risk by the age of 2 years.

Type III

Benign spinal muscular atrophy (Kugelberg–Welander disease). Most cases follow autosomal recessive inheritance, but a few isolated cases may be environmental or represent new dominant mutations[9]. Severe handicap in childhood may occur in sibs of mild cases. Offspring of affected individuals will usually be normal.

Myasthenia Gravis

In the usual adult form genetic risks are extremely low; in one series of over 400 patients, one pair of affected sibs were the only familial cases[10]. Transient congenital myasthenia gravis is seen in about 20 per cent of the offspring of affected mothers, but unlike the corresponding situation in myotonic dystrophy, does not produce permanent disease. The only group showing a clear genetic basis is the rare form with onset in infancy, which appears to be autosomal recessive[11]. It is of interest that an association has been found between myasthenia gravis and the HLA antigen DRw3 and B8 (*see Table* 3.4, p. 54). This is a good illustration of the fact that such associations do *not* prove that a disease is predominantly genetic in its causation.

Möbius' Syndrome

This diagnosis is frequently misapplied to children with other myopathies or anterior horn cell disorders presenting with facial and ocular palsies. If these can be excluded, the recurrence risk is probably low.

Peroneal Muscular Atrophy (Charcot–Marie–Tooth Disease)

This group links the hereditary neuropathies with the spinal muscular atrophies. All modes of inheritance have been recognized, but the majority are autosomal dominant. Nerve conduction studies allow two main groups to be distinguished[12].

Type 1 (Delayed nerve conduction). Onset is usually early with sensory loss and moderate disability. Most cases are autosomal dominant, but about 20 per cent are recessive. For an isolated case a risk of around 1 in 12 for sibs and 1 in 16 for children has been estimated[13].

Type 2 (Normal nerve conduction). Commonly late onset and benign. Inheritance is autosomal dominant in the great majority but apparently normal family members should be carefully studied to exclude subclinical disease. For isolated cases the risk is around 1 in 30 for sibs and 1 in 10 for children.

Hereditary Sensory Neuropathies and Related Disorders

These rare disorders, mostly following autosomal dominant inheritance, are rarely recognized with certainty in isolated patients. Genetic advice is better based on the pattern in an individual family rather than on predetermined rules. The group includes amyloid neuropathy, hypertrophic neuropathy, and various other types known only from a few families. The recessively inherited metabolic disorders Fabry's disease (X-linked) and Refsum's disease (autosomal recessive) may also present as neuropathies.

The uncommon sensory disorders, congenital insensitivity to pain and familial dysautonomia, both also follow autosomal recessive inheritance; the latter is almost entirely restricted to Jews.

A full classification of the hereditary neuropathies is given by White[14].

References

1. Thompson W. H. S. (1969) The biochemical identification of the carrier state in X-linked recessive (Duchenne) muscular dystrophy. *Clin. Chim. Acta* **26**, 207–221.
2. Bundey S. E., Crawley J. M., Edwards J. H. et al. (1979) Serum creatine kinase levels in pubertal, mature, pregnant and postmenopausal women. *J. Med. Genet.* **16**, 117–121.
3. Zellweger H. and Antonik A. (1975) Newborn screening for Duchenne muscular dystrophy. *Pediatrics* **55**, 30–34.
4. Gardner-Medwin D., Bundey S. and Green S. (1978) Early diagnosis of Duchenne muscular dystrophy. *Lancet* **1**, 1102.

5. Skinner R., Emery A. E. H., Anderson A. J. B. et al. (1975) The detection of carriers of benign (Becker-type) X-linked muscular dystrophy. *J. Med. Genet.* **12**, 131–134.

6. Harper P. S. (1975) Congenital myotonic dystrophy in Britain. I. Clinical aspects. *Arch. Dis. Child.* **50**, 505–513.

7. Harper P. S. (1973) Presymptomatic detection and genetic counselling in myotonic dystrophy. *Clin. Genet.* **4**, 134–140.

8. Pearn J. H., Carter C. O. and Wilson J. (1973) The genetic identity of acute infantile spinal muscular atrophy. *Brain* **96**, 463–470.

9. Pearn J. H. (1979) Segregation analysis of chronic childhood spinal muscular atrophy. *J. Med. Genet.* **15**, 418–423.

10. Herrmann C. (1965) Myasthenia gravis occurring in families. *Neurology* **15**, 267.

11. Bundey S. (1972) A genetic study of infantile and juvenile myasthenia gravis. *J. Neurol. Neurosurg. Psychiat.* **35**, 41–51.

12. Thomas P. K., Calne D. B. and Stewart G. (1974) Hereditary motor and sensory polyneuropathy (peroneal muscular atrophy). *Ann. Hum. Genet.* **38**, 111–153.

13. Harding A. and Thomas P. K. (1980) *J. Neurol. Sci.* In press.

14. White H. H. (1978) Neurology. In: Jackson L. G. and Schimke R. N. (ed.), *Medical Genetics: A Source Book for Physicians.* New York, Wiley. (Tables also reproduced in McKusick V. A. (1978) *Mendelian Inheritance in Man.* Baltimore, Johns Hopkins University Press.)

15. Sibert J. R., Harper P. S., Thompson R. J. et al. (1979) Carrier detection in Duchenne muscular dystrophy. Evidence from a study of obligatory carriers and mothers of isolated cases. *Arch. Dis. Child.* **54**, 534–537.

Further Reading

Becker P. E. (1977) *Myotonia Congenita and Syndromes associated with Myotonia.* Stuttgart, Thieme.

Dubowitz V. (1978) *Muscle Disorders in Childhood.* Philadelphia, Saunders.

Harper P. S. (1979) *Myotonic Dystrophy.* Philadelphia, Saunders.

CHAPTER TEN

Central Nervous System and Psychiatric Disorders

Four important groups of disease are covered in this chapter:

1. Chronic disorders of the central nervous system, many of them progressive and most at present untreatable.
2. Central nervous system malformations.
3. Mental retardation.
4. Behavioural disorders.

All four groups are relatively common, produce a serious burden on patients and families and are poorly understood in terms of aetiology. For these reasons, genetic counselling is of particular importance. Fortunately a large amount of careful study has been devoted to the genetic aspects of these disorders so that counselling has a firmer basis than might be expected from our ignorance of the underlying causative factors.

Huntington's Chorea

This disease, in the author's opinion, represents the largest and most difficult genetic counselling problem among the Mendelian disorders of adult life. The severe burden imposed on families by the disease and by fear of it, the present inadequacy of preventive and therapeutic measures, and the very real possibility that hasty or insensitive genetic counselling may do more harm than good, all add to the feeling of inadequacy that most of us have when attempting to grapple with this disorder.

Huntington's chorea, though regularly autosomal dominant in its inheritance, is late and very variable in its onset, and from this arise most of the difficulties. To advise an affected individual or the spouse that their children have a 50 per cent risk is arithmetically a simple (if depressing) procedure, but most individuals requiring advice are the healthy offspring themselves. At present, no proven test for the preclinical state exists and it is thus impossible to separate those who will remain healthy and whose own children will be free from risk, from those who will later develop the disease.

Despite this, the careful use of all available genetic information and a knowledge of the distribution of ages at onset can be of considerable help, as shown in *Fig.* 10.1. Although drawn up for a particular population, this curve is probably of general application. This information is especially

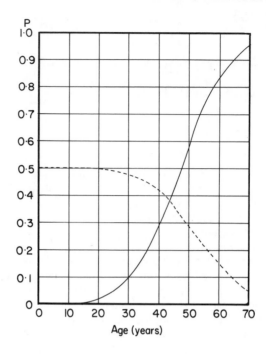

Fig. 10.1. Probability that an individual possessing the gene for HC will have developed the disorder by a certain age (from Harper et al. (1) with additional data provided by Dr Robert Newcombe).

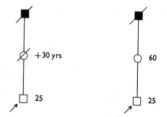

Fig. 10.2. Use of age-modified risks in Huntington's chorea.

	Prior risk	1 in 4	Prior risk	1 in 4
	Modified risk ≃ 1 in 4		Modified risk 1 in 27	

valuable where a parent at risk has died relatively young, but apparently healthy, as seen in *Fig.* 10.2.

A difficult question, not confined to Huntington's chorea, is how far ages at onset are correlated within families. The variation within a family is such that unless information is available from many members, it is better to rely on the overall curve.

Juvenile Huntington's chorea is rare, but well documented; it is almost always *paternally* transmitted (the opposite to myotonic dystrophy). It commonly presents atypically, with mental retardation and rigidity rather than chorea; chorea occurring in childhood is *unlikely* to be due to Huntington's chorea, and other conditions such as *benign hereditary chorea* (*see below*) should be considered.

Isolated Cases

Most of these prove, on careful investigation of living family members and records of previous generations, not to be isolated at all. In some cases early death of parents and lack of records makes it impossible to exclude transmission of the disease – in others paternity may be in doubt. True isolated cases are rare, but certainly exist, forming around 1 per cent of all cases in the author's experience, though a higher proportion is thought likely by some workers. If careful neurological investigation has excluded other causes of the clinical picture, the case should be accepted as a new mutation for Huntington's chorea, with a 50 per cent risk to offspring. Unfortunately, some neurologists refuse to diagnose Huntington's chorea without a positive family history – this seems as illogical as refusing to diagnose achondroplasia because the parents are healthy! Where real doubt exists, the passage of time will help to make the situation clearer.

Associated Problems

Calculating the risks is perhaps the least difficult task in the genetic counselling of families with Huntington's chorea. *Table* 10.1 lists some of the problems that arise; few have simple answers.

Table 10.1. Problems of genetic counselling in Huntington's chorea

Should all people at high risk be told of it?
At what age should information be given?
Who should give the information?
Should a register of high-risk individuals be kept?
Should genetic advice be 'directive'?
What support is required for individuals at risk?
What options exist for those deciding not to reproduce?

As to who should be told, the author believes that all adults at high risk should know before having children. Some parents protect their 'children' from the knowledge well into adult life, with long-term consequences that are often disastrous for them and result in deep family discord. An increasingly open attitude to the disease, partly due to active lay groups, seems to be decreasing this problem, but increasing mobility may be having a contrary effect in decreasing awareness of the family background.

When the information should be given will vary from family to family, but around the school leaving age is probably the best time for the subject to be raised, so that further discussion can occur when marriage is planned without this coming as a disruptive shock at this time.

It cannot be too strongly stressed that individuals at high risk for Huntington's chorea need support in order to enable them to cope with the information that they have been given. This is particularly the case when the disease is newly diagnosed in a family, or when the individuals concerned are being seen as part of an extended family investigation, rather than having actively sought advice themselves. Wherever possible, the initial information should come through a responsible family member or sympathetic family doctor, with the genetic clinic providing the opportunity for a fuller and more independent discussion. Where this is not feasible (all too often), the clinician giving advice, whether neurologist or geneticist, must ensure that support is provided. There is no substitute for an experienced social worker in this respect; any success the author may have had in this field is due largely to the availability of such a colleague.

For the increasing number of family members at high risk who decide not to reproduce, it is important to find alternatives. Prenatal diagnosis is not feasible at present, and adoption is usually ruled out. AID should be seriously considered where the husband is at risk, and the marriage a stable one.

Finally, the confidentiality of records and registers is a special problem in Huntington's chorea, as the information may be exceedingly damaging to prospects for career or insurance. Such information must be severely restricted to those clinicians directly involved with the family; access by administrators, community health staff, schools and other well-meaning bodies should not be allowed without the specific consent of the individual concerned.

Despite the warnings expressed in the above paragraphs the author remains optimistic about the prospects for long-term prevention of Huntington's chorea. Most cases are transmitted and so the people at risk can be identified. Recent biochemical progress gives real hope for predictive and prenatal tests in the future, and provides an incentive to active genetic counselling for families with this disease [1, 2]. Preliminary experience with systematic genetic counselling in South Wales for an entire population of high-risk family members suggests that the future incidence of the disorder can indeed be reduced (see Chapter 24).

Multiple Sclerosis

Familial occurrence (not necessarily genetic) is well documented, but uncommon. The risk to first-degree relatives is around 1 per cent and even monozygotic twin pairs are usually discordant. In the rare families in which parent and child are both affected, risks are considerably increased (around 10 per cent for subsequent children). An association with HLA DRW2 antigen exists, but it is likely that the major aetiological factors will prove to be immunological and possibly infective.

Syringomyelia
Recurrence in a family is exceptional.

Parkinson's Disease
All too often the author has found that a family history of 'Parkinson's disease' in past generations has turned out to be Huntington's chorea. This is probably due more to well-meaning attempts to play down the genetic aspects of the latter than to true diagnostic confusion.

Most cases of Parkinson's disease are idiopathic rather than secondary to arteriosclerosis or encephalitis, and a prevalence of around 1 in 10 000 is seen in most European countries. Many individual family aggregations have been reported, but most cases are sporadic. Based on the study of Mjönes in Sweden[3] a risk of around 12 per cent to first-degree relatives seems probable — whether this is best explained by action of an autosomal dominant gene with penetrance around 25 per cent or by polygenic inheritance is perhaps a matter of semantics. No presymptomatic tests or genetic associations have yet been found.

Other Involuntary Movement Disorders
'Essential tremor' is a common and benign disorder, inherited as a late onset autosomal dominant, and important mainly to distinguish it from other movement disorders. At the other extreme of life are several benign dominantly inherited tremors of head and chin beginning in infancy.

Torsion dystonia in childhood may follow autosomal dominant or autosomal recessive forms[4], the latter making up one-third of cases, and being commoner in Ashkenazic Jews. Since the forms cannot be distinguished, the risk to sibs of an isolated case is around 10 per cent. Most adult onset cases appear to be sporadic.

Hereditary benign chorea is characterized by non-progressive chorea present from infancy, without mental deterioration. Inheritance is autosomal dominant, with reduced penetrance in females. It is most important not to confuse this benign condition with Huntington's chorea[5].

Familial paroxysmal choreo-athetosis shows intermittent symptoms, as its name implies. It is autosomal dominant.

Narcolepsy
A recent study[6] has confirmed earlier impressions of Mendelian inheritance. Risks are close to those expected for autosomal dominance, being around 40 per cent for offspring of an affected patient. The risk for sibs of an isolated case is considerably less (14 per cent).

The Hereditary Ataxias
Genetic heterogeneity and confused classification are probably a bigger problem here than in almost any other group of disorders. Nevertheless, careful family documentation and clinical assessment does allow correct

genetic counselling to be given in most cases even when the diagnosis remains uncertain. A full listing of the numerous different types is given in the introductory tables to McKusick (1978).

1. Hereditary ataxia forming part of a generalized syndrome. Around 50 such syndromes have been identified, many from a single family.

2. Classic Friedreich's ataxia, with absent reflexes, cardiac involvement and early onset, is autosomal recessive, and the risk for offspring of affected individuals is minimal.

3. Ataxia accompanied by upper motor neurone signs ('spastic or Marie's ataxia') is almost always autosomal dominant. The neurological features are much more variable than classic Friedreich's ataxia; in some families optic atrophy is a prominent feature. The disorder is undoubtedly heterogeneous, but a number of pathological entities may occur within a family. Close linkage with the HLA system has been shown for two families [7], but whether this applies generally is unknown. In such a family, HLA typing would allow prediction of affected members in childhood and possibly in future antenatally.

4. X-linked cerebellar ataxia. This is very rare, but well documented [8] – cases are too infrequent to affect counselling for isolated male cases of ataxia.

A number of patients will fail to fit into any of the above groups. If the particular pattern of inheritance in the family is characteristic, this should be the basis for counselling; for isolated cases it is wise to assume autosomal dominant inheritance unless there is evidence to the contrary.

Hereditary Spastic Paraplegia

This is often very benign in its course; autosomal dominant inheritance is usual, but X-linked and autosomal recessive inheritance have occurred in several families. It is impossible to exclude a high risk for offspring of an isolated case.

Senile and Presenile Dementias

These provide difficult problems in diagnosis and counselling. The possibility of Huntington's chorea being responsible for familial clusters must be considered even over the age of 70 years.

In senile dementia of unknown cause, a fourfold increase over the general age specific risks has been found to occur in both sibs and offspring of patients [9], suggesting that specific genetic factors are operating even at this late stage. While this has important implications for society, the risks to individuals are not high – around 1·5 per cent at 70 years, 5 per cent at 75 years, and 8 per cent at 80 years. It is doubtful whether many people will request or need genetic counselling for this type of problem.

The presenile dementias are a much more difficult area. Not only is a pathological diagnosis frequently absent, or inconclusive if present, but conventional views on inheritance have been rudely shaken by the demonstration that familial aggregations apparently typical of autosomal dominant inheritance may result from infective agents. A slow virus aetiology has now been firmly established for Creutzfeldt–Jakob disease and for some families with Alzheimer's disease, quite apart from the special problem of Kuru in New Guinea. A recent survey[10] has shown 15 per cent of all Creutzfeldt–Jakob cases in N. America to be familial, with sibs and two generation families equally frequent. From the practical viewpoint, however, where a case of Alzheimer's disease or Creutzfeldt–Jakob disease is isolated, the risk for sibs or children is low. In the cases where a familial aggregation does exist, the risk is much higher; where the pattern looks autosomal dominant it is probably reasonable to advise accordingly, even though the 'gene' may not be one at all!

The form of presenile dementia known as Pick's disease appears to have higher overall genetic risks than the Alzheimer type, and so far no transmissible agent has been demonstrated. A risk of 7 per cent for sibs has been estimated, and the risk for children may be similar, but there are no satisfactory data[11]. In one series 19 per cent of cases had an affected parent, but it is not justifiable to equate this with the risk for offspring since preferential ascertainment of familial cases is likely.

Migraine
The population prevalence is 5–10 per cent; risks within families are high, but as with many common characteristics it is difficult to be certain whether a single major gene is responsible. Approximate risks are:

Offspring of two affected parents	70%
Offspring of one affected parent	45%
Offspring of two unaffected parents each with affected sibs	30%

Neurofibromatosis
Inheritance is autosomal dominant, with new mutations representing 1/4 to 1/2 of all cases. Careful examination of apparently unaffected family members is essential before pronouncing them to be unaffected. The presence of six or more pigmented spots over 1·5 cm diameter and of the characteristic appearance is an indication that the gene is present, but young children frequently show only inconspicuous signs of the disorder. An observation of great interest and practical importance is that cases with severe childhood complications such as malignancy and mental retardation usually have an affected mother. Miller and Hall[12] found over half of all maternally transmitted cases to be of the most severe grade, and sibs of such cases were also severely affected. It seems possible that, as with myotonic dystrophy, the intra-uterine environment interacts adversely with the neurofibromatosis gene. Conversely it would appear that the risk of severe disease in the offspring of affected males is small.

Bilateral acoustic neuromas may occur with neurofibromatosis or as a separate, dominantly inherited abnormality.

Von Hippel–Lindau Syndrome
This disorder is characterized by haemangiomatous cysts of the retina, brain (especially cerebellum), kidney and other viscera. Inheritance is normally autosomal dominant, though one family very suggestive of recessive inheritance has been noted[13]. Penetrance may be incomplete, so apparently unaffected members should be carefully assessed before being reassured. CT scan may be helpful.

Tuberous Sclerosis[14]
This disorder follows autosomal dominant inheritance, but causes considerable problems in genetic counselling because of its variability. The classic skin lesions (multiple depigmented patches, adenoma sebaceum, subungual fibromas) may be the only abnormalities present in some patients, while others may develop epilepsy or be severely retarded from cerebral involvement. CT scan is particularly helpful in showing intraventricular lesions; skull X-ray may show calcification. The birth of a severely affected child to a mildly affected parent cannot be excluded, and since individuals who reproduce are less severely affected than average, their offspring are likely to be more severely affected than themselves.

At least two-thirds of cases appear to represent new mutations, in which case the risks of recurrence in future children will be minimal. Careful examination of such parents, including examination of the skin under UV light for depigmented patches, skull X-ray, and if doubt exists, CT scan, should be made before concluding that the case is indeed a new mutation.

Epilepsy
About one person in 20 has an epileptic attack at some time, while the prevalence of recurrent epileptic attacks is around 1 in 160 in Great Britain.

Epilepsy may be secondary to a variety of environmental or hereditary disorders. Among primary epileptic disorders most do not follow Mendelian inheritance, apart from:

a. Petit mal epilepsy. When accompanied by the typical 'spike and wave' EEG pattern this is probably controlled by a major gene following autosomal dominant inheritance. Close to 50 per cent of first-degree relatives show the EEG defect when studied in adolescence, but penetrance is much reduced in both early childhood and in adult life. Not all those with an abnormal EEG have clinical attacks.

b. Progressive myoclonic epilepsy. Specific biochemical defects account for some families previously placed in this group, but others following autosomal recessive inheritance exist where no such cause can be found.

Estimating the risk to sibs of a single child is difficult. After two affected sibs a 1 in 4 risk is likely. (*See also* infantile spasms, p. 154.)

Primary Generalized Epilepsy
Numerous surveys have been carried out, with diverging results, probably depending on the severity of disease in the patients studied and on the social attitudes at the time. Most of the studies were done between 20 and 40 years ago, and though massive in numbers, the earlier ones did not have the benefit of EEG classification. *Table* 10.2 gives the approximate risks

Table 10.2. Genetic risks in idiopathic epilepsy

Individual affected	Clinical epilepsy	Abnormal EEG
Monozygotic twin	85%	90%
Dizygotic twin	4%	30–50%
Sib	2%	
Parent	5%	10%
Two sibs	8% (approx)	
One sib + one parent	10% (approx)	
Both parents	15% (approx)	

for different classes of relative. No satisfactory figures exist for families with multiple affected members; Alstrom's series, which gave lower risks than others, showed a 5 per cent risk for sibs of a patient where a parent was also affected; this may be an underestimate. The figures for multiple cases in *Table* 10.2 are derived from what would be expected in a polygenic disorder of high frequency and moderately high heritability.

Cerebral Aneurysms
Occasional family clusters suggestive of autosomal dominant inheritance have been recorded, but in general these aneurysms are rarely familial, except when associated with polycystic kidney disease. The same is true for most cerebral angiomata (provided the von Hippel–Lindau syndrome has been excluded).

Dyslexia
There has been considerable argument as to whether a specific disorder causing reading disability actually exists, but it seems likely that it does, and that it is frequently familial. Finucci et al.[15] have made a careful study of dyslexia and have shown a pattern suggestive of autosomal dominant inheritance with reduced penetrance in females.

Cerebral Palsy
This diagnosis should be mistrusted. All too often it merely camouflages ignorance of a variety of neurological disorders (often genetic), in the same

way that the term 'amyotonia congenita' does for specific causes of the floppy infant. The question to be asked is: does sufficient evidence of perinatal anoxia, prematurity, or other factors exist to explain the observed clinical problem? If the answer is 'yes', then genetic risks are clearly negligible. If the answer is 'no', then one should ask whether sufficient investigation has been done to identify any specific primary neurological disorder. The problem lies less with newly diagnosed patients, carefully studied in a good centre than with those families where a relative in a previous generation has been labelled as 'cerebral palsy' with little or no investigation. It may be necessary to reassess the original patient if sensible counselling is to be given.

A recent British study has shown an overall recurrence risk of only 1 per cent. However, several subgroups have been noted to have a higher risk, notably congenital ataxia and symmetrical tetraplegia without definite external cause, in both of which the recurrence risk is about 10–12 per cent for sibs. The athetoid type, formerly associated strongly with kernicterus, also may have a largely genetic basis when no external factors exist.

Neural Tube Defects

Despite much work and many hypotheses, the aetiology of neural tube defects remains unknown. Their incidence varies greatly even within quite restricted geographical areas, and it is well recognized that a high proportion of affected fetuses are lost as spontaneous abortions. Indeed, it has been suggested (though not confirmed) that geographical variation in birth incidence may be due more to differences in the proportion aborted than to a true difference in incidence at conception.

Neural tube defects may occur as part of chromosomal and other severe malformation syndromes, including the recessively inherited Meckel syndrome (*see below*); there is an increased frequency in association with congenital heart disease, diaphragmatic aplasia and oesophageal atresia.

All studies agree that anencephaly and spina bifida are closely related genetically and in pathogenesis. It is essential that this is indicated to families seen for genetic counselling, since a high risk of recurrence of the invariably fatal anencephaly is acceptable to some, whereas a surviving but handicapped child with spina bifida would not be. In general, the recurrence risk is equally distributed for anencephaly and spina bifida, regardless of which the index case had.

The recurrence risks for neural tube defects are summarized in *Table 10.3*. The incidence of the disorder does not appear to influence the recurrence risk as much as might be expected, though it is likely to be 3 per cent or even less in 'low' incidence areas of Europe and America. The sex of index case or individual at risk does not appear to alter risks greatly either. It can be seen that risks are low for all except first-degree relatives, and a detectable increase in risk is not seen for a relationship more distant than first cousins.

Table 10.3. Anencephaly and spina bifida: recurrence risks

Individual affected	Risk (%)
One sib	5
Two sibs	12
One second-degree relative	
(uncle/aunt or half sib)	2
One third-degree relative	1
One parent	4

These risks are for a high incidence area such as Wales. There is some evidence (*see* Nevin N., *Lancet* **1**, 1301, 1980) that social class as well as geographical incidence may affect recurrence risk, and that it may have declined in recent years, but data are still inadequate for subdivision.

The situation for families at risk has been completely changed by the advent of prenatal diagnosis, using amniotic fluid alphafetoprotein (*see* Chapter 6). This will detect virtually all subsequent cases of anencephaly and at least 90 per cent of cases of spina bifida, those undetected being covered defects or small open ones. Thus the risk of an *undetected* neural tube defect in the offspring of a couple with one affected child (a prior risk of 1 in 20) is reduced by a normal alphafetoprotein to around 1 in 380.

The use of radioimmunoassay for maternal serum alphafetoprotein as a screening test for all pregnancies in the detection of neural tube defects is at present being evaluated in a number of centres. As discussed in Chapter 6 it seems likely to prove possible to detect about 90 per cent of cases of anencephaly and 60–80 per cent of cases of open spina bifida in this way, though the organizational and ethical problems of such an approach are considerable.

Data are now becoming available for the offspring of patients affected with spina bifida, and show a risk of around 3–4 per cent regardless of which parent is affected [16]. Amniocentesis is clearly indicated for such pregnancies. No increase in other abnormalities has been noted.

Spina Bifida Occulta

This term is applied both to individuals with spinal dysraphism, showing a significant spinal defect, usually lumbosacral and often associated with a pigmented or hairy patch of skin, and also to radiological absence of one or two vertebral arches, usually discovered incidentally following an x-ray for backache or other unrelated symptom. The first group shows an increased incidence of overt neural tube defects in their offspring and sibs, with a risk similar to that for overt spina bifida, and it is reasonable to offer amniocentesis in this situation. The second group, amounting to around 5 per cent of the general population, shows no evidence of any increased risk and it is unfortunate that the term 'spina bifida' is used at all here, as women aware that they have this variant may be seriously alarmed at the possibility of clinical spina bifida occurring in their children, Amniocentesis is not justified in view of its known risks.

Hydrocephalus

This frequently accompanies spina bifida, and a careful check should be made before assuming that hydrocephalus is an isolated and primary phenomenon. The great majority of families do not follow a Mendelian pattern; an X-linked type with aqueduct stenosis exists, but is extremely rare, and counselling as for an X-linked trait should only be given if the pedigree pattern is clearly X-linked or if the other characteristic features of this type are present. The recurrence risk of 'ordinary hydrocephalus' regardless of the precise anatomical basis is around 3 per cent after a single affected child and 8 per cent after 2 affected children. No satisfactory figures for offspring of affected individuals yet exist.

An important question is whether there is overlap with spina bifida—anencephaly, since prenatal diagnosis is possible in this group while it is not for hydrocephalus. Most studies have not shown an overlap between the two conditions in families, but a recent study of pooled data[17] has suggested that there is a small, but definite occurrence (1—2 per cent) of spina bifida—anencephaly in subsequent children born to parents of a child with hydrocephalus. This means that amniocentesis (or at least maternal blood screening for AFP) may have to be considered in pregnancies at risk for hydrocephalus, even though this will be unlikely to detect the occurrence of hydrocephalus itself. Ultrasound may well be able to detect cases of hydrocephalus in early pregnancy in the near future; early developing types with spina bifida, and the severe hydranencephaly seem particularly suitable.

Encephalocoele

This should probably be regarded as part of the anencephaly—spina bifida complex and risks given as such, though an encephalocoele itself is unlikely to be diagnosed prenatally. An important association to recognize is the autosomal recessive *Meckel's syndrome*, in which encephalocoele and hypoplasia of the olfactory lobes are accompanied by a variety of other malformations, notably cleft lip or palate, polydactyly, renal cystic disease and eye defects (coloboma, cataract, microphthalmos).

Microcephaly

This may result from a variety of intrauterine factors including congenital infections, teratogens and maternal phenylketonuria; it may also be part of many genetic malformation syndromes, including the more severe auto-somal trisomies and deletions, and is a striking feature of the autosomal recessive Seckel's syndrome (Bird-headed dwarfism). Isolated *severe* microcephaly with a normal facial structure is usually inherited as an autosomal recessive, and ultrasound monitoring should be seriously considered in a pregnancy at risk for the severe form. By contrast, other types of microcephaly with mental retardation appear to have a low recurrence risk (p. 154).

Holoprosencephaly
Here, there is failure of development of the forebrain with associated facial features. It is usually lethal. The condition may be isolated or it may be part of trisomy 13. In either case, it is normally sporadic (but *see* Meckel's syndrome, *above*).

Agenesis of Corpus Callosum
This may occur as part of a more general cerebral maldevelopment or it may be isolated; most cases have been sporadic though occasional families following an apparently X-linked recessive pattern have been recorded.

Cerebral Gigantism (Sotos' syndrome)
This poorly defined disorder is usually sporadic; a few cases of affected sibs are known, but the recurrence risk is probably low unless consanguinity or other factors suggestive of recessive inheritance are present.

Mental Retardation
For the purpose of genetic counselling, it is useful to consider mental retardation in two major categories.

1. Severe mental retardation (IQ 50 or less) Prevalence c. 3/1,000.
2. Mild mental retardation (IQ 50–70)

All IQ levels above 70 are generally considered as part of the normal range.

The importance of this division stems from the fact that mild mental retardation behaves genetically as the lower end of a normal distribution, so that the IQ levels in sibs or offspring are closely influenced by those of the parents (*see below*). By contrast in severe mental retardation parental intelligence is usually normal and a sharp discontinuity is seen between family members who are affected and the normal members, with little increase in mild retardation in between. It is also in severe mental retardation that specific causes are most likely to be found, whose accurate recognition is essential for genetic counselling.

Specific Causes of Mental Retardation
The number of specific disorders of which mental retardation is an integral or major component is exceedingly large and is growing steadily, a fact which makes it important to reassess individuals who have not received thorough investigation. Some of the disorders have been found to have a definite aetiological basis, which may be biochemical, chromosomal or environmental; in most cases the underlying cause remains unknown, but

Table 10.4. Mendelian disorders causing or frequently associated with mental retardation

---

Autosomal dominant
  Tuberous sclerosis (epiloia)
  Neurofibromatosis (not constant)
  Myotonic dystrophy (particularly early onset and congenital cases)
  Huntington's chorea (juvenile form)
  Apert's syndrome
  Mandibulofacial dysostosis (not constant)
Autosomal recessive
  Phenylketonuria
  Homocystinuria
  Galactosaemia
  Hyperammonaemias
  Neurolipidoses (including Tay–Sachs, Gaucher's, metachromatic
    leucodystrophy and numerous others)
  Mucopolysaccharidoses (types I, III)
  Wilson's disease
  Sjögren–Larsson syndrome
  Bardet–Biedl syndrome
  Microcephaly (severe form)
  Seckel's syndrome
  Carpenter's acrocephalopolysyndactyly
  Ataxia telangiectasia
  Xeroderma pigmentosum
X-linked
  Hunter's syndrome (MPS II)
  Lesch–Nyhan syndrome
  Duchenne muscular dystrophy (not constant)
  Menkes' syndrome
  Renpenning's 'non-specific' mental retardation
  Fragile X chromosome syndrome (includes some Renpenning type families)
  Lowe's oculocerebrorenal syndrome
  Norrie's disease
  Incontinentia pigmentia (male lethal, X-linked dominant)
  Albright's hereditary osteodystrophy
  Cerebral sclerosis with Addison's disease
  Cerebral sclerosis, Pelizaeus–Merzbacher type
  Orofaciodigital syndrome (male lethal, X-linked dominant)
  X-linked aqueduct stenosis
  Anhidrotic ectodermal dysplasia (occasional)

---

the occurrence of a constant series of physical abnormalities may allow the delineation of a clinical syndrome.

One major group of specific disorders to be recognized is that following Mendelian inheritance, for it is here that the risks of recurrence in sibs are highest, particularly the autosomal recessive and X-linked recessive disorders. *Table* 10.4 lists some of the major causes; many are considered in more detail in other chapters.

Among the non-Mendelian causes of mental retardation (*Table* 10.5), chromosomal disorders are particularly important to recognize. Almost all

Table 10.5. Non-Mendelian and chromosomal syndromes associated with mental retardation

---

Chromosomal (See Chapter 4)
    Down's syndrome
    Other autosomal abnormalities (numerous)
    XXY (Klinefelter) syndrome
    XXX syndrome (and other multiple X)
    XXYY syndrome
    XO (Turner) syndrome (occasional)
Non-chromosomal
    De Lange's syndrome
    Noonan's syndrome
    Sturge–Weber syndrome
    Prader–Willi syndrome
    Rubinstein–Taybi syndrome
    Hallerman–Streiff syndrome
    Congenital hypothyroidism
    Hydrocephalus and hydranencephalus
    Infantile hypercalcaemia syndrome
Environmental factors (See Chapter 23)
    Congenital infections (rubella, cytomegalovirus, toxoplasma)
    Teratogens (alcohol, phenytoin)
    Anoxia
    Brain damage associated with prematurity
    Intrauterine growth retardation syndromes
    Maternal phenylketonuria
    Trauma (non-accidental)
    Lead poisoning

---

unbalanced autosomal disorders are associated with mental retardation; in older patients said previously to have been chromosomally normal, it is worth restudying with the more sensitive banding techniques. Unless a parent also has a chromosomal rearrangement the recurrence risk will be low, and a confident prediction of clinical normality can be made for individuals shown to be normal chromosomally at amniocentesis or subsequently.

If an environmental cause can be identified, recurrence is also unlikely, provided that the harmful agent is not still operating. Caution must be made not to attribute falsely mental retardation to perinatal anoxia or other factors which may be the result of the underlying disorder rather than its cause.

The less frequent association of mental retardation with a large number of specific physical syndromes is of extreme importance in genetic counselling, for many couples who would accept the risk of physical handicap in an affected child are unwilling to accept the additional risk of mental handicap. Unfortunately, bias of ascertainment or reporting often makes the frequency of mental retardation difficult to assess. Histidinaemia, anhidrotic ectodermal dysplasia, Duchenne and myotonic dystrophy are but a few examples.

Severe Non-specific Mental Retardation

Despite the most careful study, the majority of severely mentally retarded children have no clear underlying causative factor or associated syndrome, and no relevant pedigree information. Here one is forced to use the general empiric recurrence risks, even though many such cases are likely to prove in the future to have their own specific basis. Fortunately, a number of studies have been carried out, with broadly similar results; one of the first systematic studies was that of Penrose[18]; Davison[19] concentrated on X-linked mental retardation, while Bundey and Carter[20] analysed referrals to the Hospital for Sick Children, London, who had been intensively investigated, though they do not represent an unselected population. The overall reccurrence risk to sibs appears to be a little under 3 per cent (i.e. about 10 X the population risk); the somewhat higher risk to male sibs in some series probably results from a generally greater susceptibility of males as well as from inclusion of X-linked families (*see below*). *Table* 10.6 gives approximate risks suitable for counselling.

Table 10.6. Genetic risks in severe 'non-specific' mental retardation (I.Q. 50 or less) (based on Penrose, Davison, and Bundey and Carter)

Affected	Individual at risk	Risk	
Isolated case,	Sib (both sexes)	1 in 35	
male or female	Male sib	1 in 25	
	Female sib	1 in 50	
Two sibs, regardless	Sib of either sex	1 in 4	
of sex			
Isolated case M or F			
Parents consanguineous	Sib of either sex	1 in 7	
Affected male with	Male sib	1 in 2 ⎫	X-linkage
affected maternal uncle	Female sib	low ⎭	probable
One affected parent	Child of either		
(either sex)	sex	1 in 10	
One affected parent +	Child of either		
affected child	sex	1 in 5	
Two affected parents	Child of either sex	1 in 2	

Additional family information may modify the risk estimate. Thus consanguinity in the parents increases the likelihood of autosomal recessive inheritance and Penrose found a risk of 1 in 7 for sibs of such cases. Davison advised a risk of 1 in 4 on the basis that autosomal recessive inheritance is most likely in the presence of consanguinity; however, polygenic inheritance is also affected by consanguinity so there seems no reason to abandon the observed figures found by Penrose. Where two affected sibs exist, a risk of close to 1 in 4 to future sibs is appropriate, regardless of sex, unless a pattern suggesting X linkage is present in previous generations.

Risks to offspring of affected individuals are not a significant problem in severe mental retardation; no estimate of risk can be deduced from the rare examples of reproduction in such cases. The risk to second-degree relatives, i.e. the offspring of healthy individuals who have a mentally retarded sib or sibs, is a considerable worry. This is especially the case where a healthy woman has a retarded brother or brothers, a situation in which the possibility of X-linked inheritance must be seriously considered. If a maternally related affected male is present in a previous genetation, this is strong support for X-linkage. Where the affected individuals are female, or of both sexes, an X-linked recessive basis can be discounted, and risks for second-degree relatives are small. Third-degree relatives are unlikely to be at significant risk unless the family pattern is clearly X-linked.

X-linked Mental Retardation (Renpenning's Syndrome)

While the male excess in mental retardation can partly be explained by increased male vulnerability to adverse environmental factors, there is no doubt that an X-linked gene or genes play a considerable part in 'non-specific' moderate to severe mental retardation. In Davison's study[19] there was a pedigree pattern suggestive of X-linkage in 8 out of 141 families, while the number of families with only males affected was twice that with only females affected.

Families showing an X-linked pedigree pattern do not show consistent phenotypic differences from others except for the presence of macrorchidism in some affected males; the degree of retardation is frequently moderate rather than severe; carrier females do not show any abnormalities. Recently some families have been found to be associated with a hereditary fragile site on the X chromosome and it has been suggested that this chromosomal defect may actually be causative for the mental retardation[21]. If this proves to be a consistent finding it will be of considerable importance since the defect might be detected prenatally in fetal blood (it is not seen in cultured cells) and in carriers. However, it is not yet known what proportion of individuals showing the defect are clinically abnormal, nor what proportion of X-linked mental retardation can be accounted for by it.

Before non-specific X-linked mental retardation is accepted as a diagnosis, special care must be taken to exclude other X-linked syndromes accompanied by mental retardation, notably the Lesch—Nyhan syndrome, the Hunter syndrome (MPS II) and X-linked hydrocephalus.

Other Specific Groups in 'Non-specific' Mental Retardation

In addition to families showing X-linked inheritance there are other groups with sufficient distinguishing features to give risk figures different from those in *Table* 10.6. A particular high risk group noted by Bundey and Carter and by others previously is that of symmetrical spasticity with mental retardation; here the recurrence in sibs seems to be around 10 per cent. By contrast they found an extremely low recurrence risk for other forms of 'cerebral palsy' associated with mental retardation, though it should be noted that this was an intensively investigated series in which the term cerebral palsy was likely to be restricted to cases with clear evidence of anoxia (see p. 146).

Another important low risk subgroup is that of idiopathic infantile spasms; Bundey and Carter found no recurrence here except when associated with spasticity. A similar low risk was found for mental retardation associated with microcephaly. This contrasts with the autosomal recessive inheritance of the specific type of severe microcephaly with normal facial structure.

Mild Mental Retardation

It has already been stated that in contrast to severe mental retardation, mild mental retardation behaves as part of the normal distribution of intelligence, as a polygenic trait. One or both parents are commonly retarded, and the intelligence of future children will be distributed around the mid-parental mean. Correspondingly the risk of an intelligent couple having a further mildly retarded child is low.

Nevertheless, a careful search should be made for specific causes that may underly mild mental retardation, and which if found may radically alter the genetic risks.

Normal Intelligence

When faced with an enquiry about the inheritance of normal intelligence, the initial reaction of the physician, daily seeing patients with inherited causes of severe mental and physical handicap, is to tell parents to be content with the fact that their child is normal. Nevertheless, intelligence is undeniably an attribute of the highest importance and is not so completely under the control of the environment as some would wish to believe. Adoption agencies recognize this when they try to 'match' children with prospective parents.

The following general comments may be helpful in answering questions from families:

1. The mating pattern is highly assortative for intelligence, i.e. intelligent people tend to marry each other and likewise for the less intelligent.

2. On average the intelligence of a child is likely to be midway between that of the parents, with a considerable scatter around this mean.

3. It is possible for the intelligence of a child to be outside the limits of the parents; the greater the departure from the mean, the less likely will this be.

4. Too much reliance should not be placed on the results of single IQ tests, especially in early childhood. One of the author's patients with Marfan's syndrome, initially investigated in infancy for 'mental retard-

ation', is currently studying astrophysics after winning scholarships to three separate universities!

Schizophrenia

When strict diagnostic criteria are used (there is close agreement on these over most of Western Europe, but not in N. America) the risk of anyone developing the disorder during his lifetime is close to 1 per cent. Numerous studies have shown a strong familial tendency, and that this is principally genetic is suggested by studies of monozygotic twins reared apart[22]. There has been considerable argument as to whether the basis of inheritance is a single major gene, modified by other factors, or whether a polygenic model is more appropriate; the subject is fully discussed by Slater and Cowie, but it is doubtful whether it will be resolved until we know more about the specific biochemical basis of the disorder.

The seriousness of the disease and its high prevalence make schizophrenia a major genetic counselling problem. Numerous surveys have been done on the risks to relatives, with wide variation in results. *Table* 10.7

Table 10.7. Genetic risks in schizophrenia (based on Slater and Cowie, 1971)

Affected relative	Risk (%)
Sib	9
Parent	13
Sib + one parent	15
Both parents	40
Second-degree relative	3
Monozygotic twin	40
Dizygotic twin	10

gives approximate risk figures; it can be seen that the risks are considerable for all first-degree relatives. Several additional points need to be considered in counselling.

1. The risk to offspring has been shown to be less in the milder and later onset paranoid and simple schizophrenic states than in the hebephrenic and catatonic types.

2. In addition to the occurrence of classic schizophrenia in relatives, there is an increased frequency of borderline psychiatric states of doubtful classification.

3. There is a slight increase of schizophrenia in the sibs of patients with other types of psychosis, but in general schizophrenia appears to be genetically distinct, particularly when diagnostic difficulties are allowed for.

4. Care must be taken to exclude other primary disorders which may present with features suggestive of schizophrenia and which may follow Mendelian inheritance, e.g. homocystinuria, Huntington's chorea.

Affective Psychoses

These, like schizophrenia, represent a major problem in the community. The expectation of developing a major manic-depressive psychosis in a person's lifetime is around 1 per cent, but if milder depressive states are included, the figure may be as high as 5 per cent and is rising. There seems to be a clear genetic distinction among classic affective psychoses into those that are unipolar, i.e. characterized by depression only, and those that are bipolar, i.e. characterized by alternating mania and depression. The risk to relatives appears also to be higher where the proband has early onset than when onset is later (over 40 years).

Table 10.8 summarizes the main risk categories. It should be stressed that different surveys have given a wide range of estimates. Where age at

Table 10.8. Overall genetic risks in affective psychoses

	Risk (%)
Sibs	13
Children	15
Monozygotic twin	70
Dizygotic twin	20
Second-degree relatives	5
First cousins	3·5

onset in the proband is known, the risk to first-degree relatives should probably be increased to 20 per cent when onset was under 40 years, and reduced to 10 per cent when onset was over 40 years.

Behavioural Disorders

When the major psychoses have been excluded one is left with a number of disorders where classification and aetiology are much less clear-cut, and where there is much argument over the relative importance of genetic and environmental factors. (These include obsessive-compulsive neuroses, anxiety states, homosexuality and hysteria.) A considerable amount of data from family and twin studies does exist, but it is not really suitable for use in genetic counselling. The high frequency of many of these traits in the population and the lack of clear distinction from normality are further difficulties.

Other problems where the possibility of a genetic basis has been suggested are criminality and alcoholism. The relationship of the former with the XYY syndrome remains debatable (*see* Chapter 4); in alcoholism a genetic basis, possibly related to biochemical polymorphisms in metabolism of alcohol, seems likely, but is extremely difficult to separate from environmental factors.

References
1. Harper P. S., Walker D. A., Tyler A. et al. (1979) Huntington's chorea. The basis for long term prevention. *Lancet* 2, 346–349.
2. Harper P. S., Walker D. A., Tyler A. et al. (1980) Huntington's chorea. Evidence for reduction in future incidence associated with systematic genetic counselling (in press).
3. Mjönes H. (1949) Paralysis agitans: a clinical and genetic study. *Acta Psychiat. Scand.* Suppl. 54, 1–195.
4. Bundey S., Harrison M. J. G. and Marsden C. D. (1975) A genetic study of torsion dystonia. *J. Med. Genet.* 12, 12–19.
5. Harper P. S. (1978) Benign hereditary chorea: Clinical and genetic aspects. *Clin. Genet.* 13, 85–95.
6. Baraitser M. and Parkes J. D. (1978) Genetic study of narcoleptic syndrome. *J. Med. Genet.* 15, 254–257.
7. Jackson J. F., Currier R. D., Terasaki P. I. et al. (1977) Spinocerebellar ataxia and HLA linkage. Risk prediction by HLA typing. *N. Engl. J. Med.* 296, 1138–1141.
8. Shokeir M. H. K. (1970) X-linked cerebellar ataxia. *Clin. Genet.* 1, 225–231.
9. Larsson T., Sjögren T. and Jacobson G. (1963) Senile dementia: a clinical, sociomedical and genetic study. *Acta Neurol. Scand.* Suppl. 167, 1–259.
10. Masters C. L., Harris J. O., Gajdusek D. C. et al. (1979) Creutzfeldt–Jakob disease: patterns of worldwide occurrence and the significance of familial and sporadic clustering. *Ann. Neurol.* 5, 177–188.
11. Sjögren T., Sjögren H. and Lindgren A. G. H. (1952) Morbus Alzheimer and Morbus Pick. A genetic, clinical and patho-anatomical study. *Acta Psychiat. Scand.* Suppl. 82, 1–152.
12. Miller M. and Hall J. G. (1978) Possible maternal effect on severity of neurofibromatosis. *Lancet* 2, 1071–1073.
13. Shokeir M. H. K. (1970) Von Hippel–Lindau syndrome. A report on three kindreds. *J. Med. Genet.* 7, 155–157.
14. Gomez M. R. (ed.) (1979) *Tuberous Sclerosis.* New York, Raven Press.
15. Finucci J. M., Guthrie J. T., Childs A. L. et al. (1976) The genetics of specific reading disability. *Ann. Hum. Genet.* 40, 1–23.
16. Carter C. O. and Evans K. (1973) Children of adult survivors with spina bifida cystica. *Lancet* 2, 924–926.
17. Cohen T., Stern E. and Rosenmann A. (1979) Sib risk of neural tube defect: is prenatal diagnosis indicated following the birth of a hydrocephalic child? *J. Med. Genet.* 16, 14–16.
18. Penrose L. S. (1972) *The Biology of Mental Defect.* London, Sidgwick & Jackson.
19. Davison B. C. C. (1973) Genetic studies in mental subnormality. I. Familial idiopathic severe subnormality: the question of a contribution by X-linked genes. *Br. J. Psychiat.* Special publication No. 8, 1–60.
20. Bundey S. and Carter C. O. (1974) Recurrence risks in severe undiagnosed mental deficiency. *J. Ment. Defic. Res.* 18, 115–134.
21. Sutherland G. R. (1977) Fragile sites on human chromosomes: demonstration of their dependence on the type of tissue culture medium. *Science* 197, 265–266.
22. Shields J. (1962) Monozygotic twins brought up apart and brought up together. London, Oxford University Press.

Further Reading

Chase T. N., Wexler N. and Barbeau A. (Ed.) (1979) *Huntington's Disease. Advances in Neurology.* Vol. 23. New York, Raven Press.
Gellis S. S. and Feingold (1968) *Atlas of Mental Retardation Syndromes.* Washington D.C., US Dept. of Health, Education and Welfare.

McKusick V. A. (1978) *Mendelian Inheritance in Man.* Baltimore, Johns Hopkins University Press.
The introductory tables as well as the detailed entries are especially helpful with rare and confusing neurological disorders.
Penrose L. S. (1972) *The Biology of Mental Defect.* London, Sidgwick & Jackson.
Pratt R. T. C. (1967) *Genetics of Neurological Disorders.* London, Oxford University Press.
Slater E. and Cowie V. (1971) *The Genetics of Mental Disorders.* London, Oxford University Press.

CHAPTER ELEVEN

Disorders of Bone and Connective Tissue

Primary Bone Dysplasias

Genetic counselling in this confusing group of disorders requires special care. Full X-rays and clinical assessment are essential for a firm diagnosis to be reached; even so, many cases remain undiagnosed. In such a situation, one must be guided by the pedigree pattern of the individual family; most types follow Mendelian inheritance, but for an isolated case it is often impossible to distinguish between a new dominant mutation and autosomal recessive inheritance. Few clinicians see many cases of bone dysplasia, so it is unreasonable to expect familiarity with every type. Pooling experience is a great help; the author has had fruitful associations with bone dysplasia groups in Cardiff and Bristol, and there is no doubt that the discussion of problem cases at such meetings has allowed an accurate diagnosis and genetic counselling that would not have been possible otherwise.

A special effort should be made to get photographic and X-ray evidence on all skeletal dysplasias, particularly on stillbirths. It is both surprising and frustrating how often such vital diagnostic information is not obtained or, in the case of X-rays, is destroyed by hospitals. Even old family photographs can be of great value in the case of members no longer living.

Individuals with different (or even the same) forms of dwarfism commonly marry each other, with confusing results in the offspring. Interaction of the genes is to be expected only if the disorders are allelic. The birth of a child of normal stature to such a couple may be unexpected and even pose a difficult problem for them. Many such couples are anxious to adopt children who will also be of short stature, and this should be encouraged. Obstetric difficulties in women owing to the small pelvis must not be forgotten.

Table 11.1 summarizes the inheritance of some of the major types of bone dysplasia based on the 'Paris classification'. The books of Spranger et al. and by Beighton provide clear and well illustrated diagnostic aids. Special points on some of the disorders are mentioned briefly below.

Achondroplasia

Never accept this diagnosis without checking, especially when made by an orthopaedic surgeon or an obstetrician! The case record of one stillborn infant seen personally consisted of one word – 'achondroplasia' – but

Table 11.1. Inheritance of bone dysplasias (less frequent alternatives in brackets)

Autosomal dominant
　Achondroplasia
　Hypochondroplasia
　Pseudoachondroplasia (AR)
　Dyschondrosteosis
　Osteopoikilosis
　Spondylo-epiphyseal dysplasia congenita
　Multiple epiphyseal dysplasia
　Metaphyseal dysplasia, Schmidt type
　Congenital bowing (Blount's disease)
　Cranio-metaphyseal dysplasia (AR)
　Craniocarpotarsal dysplasia (Freeman–Sheldon syndrome)
　Cleidocranial dysplasia
　Diaphyseal aclasis (multiple hereditary exostoses)
　Progressive diaphyseal dysplasia (AR)
　Nail-patella syndrome
　Fibrodysplasia ossificans progressiva (myositis ossificans)
　Trichorhinophalangeal dysplasia

Autosomal recessive
　Diastrophic dwarfism
　Metatropic dwarfism
　Achondrogenesis
　Sclerosteosis
　Pycnodysostosis
　Van Buchem's disease (most families)
　Familial metaphyseal dysplasia
　Metaphyseal dysplasia, Jansen type
　Cartilage hair hypoplasia
　Chondro-ectodermal dysplasia (Ellis–van Creveld)
　Ollier's osteochondromatosis
　Jeune's thoracic dysplasia
　Hypophosphatasia (infantile)
　Mucopolysaccharidoses (except type II)
　Weill–Marchesani syndrome
　Seckel's syndrome (Bird-headed dwarfism)

X-linked
　Spondyloepiphyseal dysplasia tarda (recessive)
　Orofaciodigital dysplasia, type I (dominant, lethal in male)
　Vitamin D resistant rickets (intermediate)
　Mucopolysaccharidosis II (recessive)
　Otopalatodigital syndrome (probably intermediate)

Variable or uncertain
　Thanatophoric dwarfism (*see* p. 162; risk to sibs around 5%)
　Chondrodysplasia punctata (*see* p. 162)
　Silver's syndrome (mostly sporadic)
　Unclassified spondyloepiphyseal dysplasias
　De Lange's syndrome (*see* p. 170; risk to sibs around 2%)
　Caffey's infantile cortical hyperostosis
　Albright's fibrous dysplasia (almost always sporadic)
　Paget's disease (probably autosomal dominant with incomplete penetrance)
　Melorheostosis (usually sporadic)

prove to be thanatophoric dwarfism. True achondroplasia rarely causes problems in neonatal life, though it can be recognized at birth; most fatal cases of 'achondroplasia' are other dysplasias. Inheritance is invariably autosomal dominant, but around 80 per cent of cases are new mutations, with no significant recurrence risk for future sibs. Homozygous achondroplasia occurs in 1/4 of the children of two achondroplastic parents and is lethal soon after birth. Another 1/4 of the children of such couples are normal.

The milder disorder *hypochondroplasia* is probably allelic to achondroplasia, since 'compounds' have been recorded when one parent has achondroplasia, the other hypochondroplasia[1]. Although most patients with hypochondroplasia have few physical problems and are mentally entirely normal, a small number of cases with mental retardation have been reported, which are probably not due to coincidence.

Pseudoachondroplasia

Both autosomal recessive and autosomal dominant forms exist, but the latter are much the more common. Thus for an isolated case with typical features and no consanguinity, the risk of offspring of affected individuals is close to 50 per cent, while the risk to sibs is low (around 3 per cent).

Spondylo-epiphyseal Dysplasias and Spondylometaphyseal Dysplasias

This group is particularly heterogeneous and confusing, a situation worsened by the tendency to place any dysplasia one cannot diagnose in this category. However, the X-linked *'tarda'* form should be clearly recognizable, even in an isolated case, by the characteristic X-ray appearance of the spine with a central 'hump' of bone, and relatively normal distal limb bones.

The severe *spondylo-epiphyseal dysplasia congenita* is frequently confused with the Morquio syndrome (mucopolysaccharidosis IV) and may follow autosomal dominant or rarely recessive inheritance. Retinal detachment is an important complication.

Dyschondrosteosis and Madelung's Deformity

Most cases of Madelung's deformity of the wrist are part of the mild, but generalized dysplasia, dyschondrosteosis, following autosomal dominant inheritance.

Multiple Epiphyseal Dysplasia

Mildly affected individuals may have only moderately reduced stature and the pattern of autosomal dominant inheritance characteristic of most families may be missed as a result. This disorder must be excluded when giving genetic advice to patients with bilateral Perthes' disease.

Chondrodystrophia Punctata (Conradi's disease)

Cataract, mental retardation and ichthyosis may all occur. Both autosomal dominant and recessive forms exist (the latter more severe). A phenocopy is also produced by maternal warfarin ingestion in early pregnancy[2], and must be excluded before a genetic basis is assumed.

Lethal Newborn Dysplasias

The major causes are listed in *Table* 11.2. Some are invariably fatal, others not so. It may be possible to recognize cases in late pregnancy by X-ray (but not early). No other prenatal diagnostic tests are available though ultrasonic measurement of limb length is under assessment. It is doubtful whether fetoscopy will be sufficiently sensitive to provide reliable detection. X-ray should always be done on a stillbirth suspected of falling in this

Table 11.2 Frequently lethal newborn bone dysplasias

Type	Inheritance
Thanatophoric dwarfism	Uncertain
Achondrogenesis (two types)	Autosomal recessive
Ellis–van Creveld syndrome	Autosomal recessive
Thoracic dysplasia (Jeune)	Autosomal recessive
Chondrodysplasia punctata (Conradi)	Usually autosomal recessive (but *see above*)
Metatropic dwarfism	Autosomal recessive
Hypophosphatasia (severe type)	Autosomal recessive
Osteogenesis imperfecta congenita	Uncertain; *see* p. 165

group since specific diagnosis may be impossible without it. Osteogenesis imperfecta congenita can be easily mistaken for a lethal newborn dysplasia. All the conditions seem to follow Mendelian inheritance, but for thanatophoric dwarfism the recurrence risk is too low for autosomal recessive inheritance yet too high for all cases to be new mutations. It is likely that heterogeneity will be demonstrated to account for this; in the meantime, the approximate recurrence risk of thanatophoric dwarfism in sibs is 5 per cent[3].

Osteopetrosis

A number of conditions are characterized by increased bone density, including pycnodysostosis, sclerosteosis and van Buchem's disease, but true osteopetrosis exists in two forms – a mild form, often asymptomatic, following autosomal dominant inheritance, and a severe childhood form with bone marrow involvement, which is autosomal recessive.

Multiple Exostoses (Diaphyseal Aclasis)

This follows a classic autosomal dominant pattern, though some individuals have only a few lesions which may not be symptomatic. By contrast *endo-*

chromatosis (Ollier's disease) is rarely transmitted to children and is of uncertain inheritance.

Limb Defects

It is impossible to deal with all the different types here; the books of Beighton, Temtamy and McKusick and Wynne-Davies should be consulted for details. A high proportion of bilateral abnormalities follow Mendelian inheritance; many form part of more general syndromes. Unilateral defects, by contrast, are usually non-genetic. Recognition of the mode of inheritance has become of particular importance recently because fetoscopy may be an appropriate preventive measure in those disorders where the clinical features are severe, the limb defect is constant and there is a high risk of recurrence. It is equally important that pregnancies where these conditions do not apply are *not* exposed to this high risk procedure.

Polydactyly

Isolated postaxial polydactyly is a harmless but common (especially in Blacks) autosomal dominant condition, showing incomplete penetrance. Important conditions with polydactyly include trisomy 13, Ellis–van Creveld and Jeune's syndromes and the Laurence–Moon–Biedl syndrome.

Syndactyly

The Poland syndrome of unilateral syndactyly and pectoral muscle aplasia is an important form to recognize since it appears to be non-genetic, possibly related to abortifacients[4]. Bilateral isolated syndactyly of hands and/or feet has several forms, all autosomal dominant. Important syndromes include the orofaciodigital syndrome (X-linked dominant, lethal in the male) and the acrocephaly-syndactylies (*see* Chapter 12).

Brachydactyly

Various distinct types exist. Inheritance is generally autosomal dominant. Syndrome associations include pseudohypoparathyroidism (X-linked dominant) and Turner's syndrome.

Ectrodactyly (split hand or lobster claw defect)

Most isolated bilateral cases follow autosomal dominant inheritance. A number of families exist in which multiple affected sibs born to healthy parents have gone on to have affected children themselves[5]. Autosomal recessive inheritance or lack of penetrance seem unsatisfactory explanations and it is likely that germinal mosaicism, 'premutation', or some other unusual genetic mechanism is operating. Whatever the cause, it means that affected individuals have a high risk of affected children even if the family pattern does appear to be autosomal recessive. An important syndrome to recognize is the EEC (ectrodactyly–ectodermal dysplasia– cleft lip and palate) syndrome, also autosomal dominant.

Limb Reduction Defects

These may be extremely difficult to distinguish. Some, in particular unilateral defects associated with 'amniotic constriction bands' are likely to be non-genetic. Other asymmetric defects may be associated with oesophageal, anal, cardiac, renal and vertebral abnormalities (the VATER association); again recurrence risk is low. Thalidomide was previously a major cause, but no other definite drug-induced defects of this type are known. New cases of thalidomide type deformity (sometimes termed 'pseudothalidomide' or Roberts' syndrome) are likely to follow autosomal recessive inheritance.

Important and variable syndromes affecting mainly the upper limbs include the following:

Thrombocytopenia—absent radius syndrome (TAR)	Autosomal recessive
Fanconi's pancytopenia	Autosomal recessive
Holt—Oram syndrome (heart-hand)	Autosomal dominant
Poland's syndrome (unilateral, with absence of pectoralis muscle)	Negligible recurrence risk
Orofaciodigital syndrome (2 types)	X-linked dominant, lethal in male. *See* p. 177

Early prenatal diagnosis of the TAR syndrome by fetal radiology has recently been shown to be feasible[6], while chromosomal instability of cultured amniotic cells may allow prenatal diagnosis of the Fanconi pancytopenia; these and ultrasound may prove to be alternatives to fetoscopy.

Connective Tissue Disorders

Osteogenesis Imperfecta

Osteogenesis imperfecta is almost certainly a heterogeneous disorder. So far the clinical and genetic classification is unsatisfactory and our biochemical knowledge has not reached the stage of allowing clear distinction between the types (*Table* 11.3). From the practical aspect of genetic counselling the following points need attention:

1. In the late onset 'tarda' forms, autosomal dominant inheritance is the rule. The occasional recessively inherited instances have mostly been in inbred populations.

2. Careful examination of apparently unaffected members is essential in mildly affected families to exclude minor manifestations, such as hearing loss (of otosclerotic type) and dentine changes, particularly where a new mutation is suspected.

3. Blue sclerae are common in healthy infants.

4. Where a severely affected infant with the 'congenita' type is born to healthy parents, most cases are sporadic and probably represent new dominant mutations. Instances of more than one such child born to healthy parents are rare, but do exist; most have been of the 'thick-bone' type on X-ray. Despite a recent study from Australia[7] UK data indicate

Table 11.3. Osteogenesis imperfecta. A provisional classification

---

1. Tarda
    a. Autosomal dominant – the great majority of cases. Severity very
          variable; almost certainly genetically heterogeneous
    b. Autosomal recessive – extremely rare. Severe course with
          progressive deformity
2. Congenita
    a. Sporadic – presumably new dominant mutations. The majority of
          cases
    b. Autosomal recessive. Rare. Bones usually thick on X-ray, with
          beaded ribs

---

that such recessive cases probably represent less than 10 per cent of the
total 'congenita' cases, so that the recurrence risk in sibs is unlikely to
exceed 3 per cent[8]. Even when the affected child does have the 'thick
bone' type, it is probable that the risk of recurrence is considerably less
than the 1 in 4 risk expected for autosomal recessive inheritance.

5. Prediction of severity of disease in the offspring of an affected
patient is difficult, but it seems clear that the risk of severe osteogenesis
imperfecta congenita is very small. Where there are sufficient affected
family members to give a guide to severity, one can be rather more confident in one's prediction.

Marfan's Syndrome

This disorder tends to be overdiagnosed in tall individuals of slender
habitus but with no cardinal signs; there is rarely doubt when the presence
or absence of the various major features is considered as a whole. Inheritance is autosomal dominant; the occurrence of major aortic complications
is unpredictable and many patients live a relatively normal life until a
sudden demise occurs. This is relevant for genetic counselling since, in the
author's experience, most patients wish for and have families. Several
patients have been of unusually high intelligence and have contributed
more in their short life than most of us will in a full span! Around half the
patients appear to be new mutations; penetrance is probably full but
apparently healthy members should be carefully checked (including
slit-lamp examination for minor degrees of lens dislocation). Care should
be taken to distinguish homocystinuria (autosomal recessive) and patients
with isolated lens dislocation due to spherophakia who happen by chance
to be tall and thin.

Ehlers–Danlos Syndrome

This group of disorders, in which hypermobility of skin and joints, skin
fragility and bruising, and rarer vascular, visceral and ocular complications
are the main features, is extremely heterogeneous. *Table* 11.4 is reproduced
from Beighton. Autosomal dominant inheritance is much the most com-

Table 11.4. The Ehlers–Danlos syndromes (after Beighton, 1978)

Type	Basic Defect	Inheritance
I	Unknown	Autosomal dominant
II	Unknown	Autosomal dominant
III	Unknown	Autosomal dominant
IV	Deficient type II collagen	Autosomal recessive or autosomal dominant
V	Lysyl oxidase deficiency	X-linked recessive
VI	Procollagen lysyl hydroxylase deficiency	Autosomal recessive
VII	Procollagen protease deficiency	Autosomal recessive

mon. Pregnancy may be dangerous in the severe forms. There is a tendency to label any new and undelineated connective tissue disorder as 'type N + 1' of the Ehlers–Danlos syndrome. Undoubtedly developments in collagen biochemistry will help identify some of these new disorders.

Cutis Laxa
This may follow either autosomal recessive or autosomal dominant inheritance so a high risk for offspring of an isolated case cannot be excluded.

Pseudoxanthoma Elasticum
Most cases follow autosomal recessive inheritance, but a few dominantly inherited families have been described, mostly with milder clinical features [9]. Asymptomatic individuals may be detected by the presence of angioid streaks in the retina.

Mucopolysaccharidoses
All types follow autosomal recessive inheritance except for type II (Hunter's syndrome). The enzymatic basis of the major types is well defined (except for Morquio's syndrome, type IV), and should be established to allow appropriate prenatal diagnosis, which is feasible for all types except type IV. Clinical distinction between male cases of type I and II and types II and III is not always easy.

Risks for offspring of healthy sibs are very small except for the X-linked type II. Carrier detection in type II is feasible using cloned fibroblast culture, but is extremely difficult; recent studies of hair bulbs are encouraging[10]. It is probably wise for all females at high risk of being type II carriers to have pregnancies monitored by fetal sexing and direct biochemical studies to distinguish affected from unaffected males. The relevant enzyme (iduronate sulphatase) is one of the few that can be measured reliably in amniotic fluid supernatant as well as in cultured cells.

The various forms of *mucolipidoses,* all exceedingly rare, follow autosomal recessive inheritance.

Arthritis and Arthropathies

The commoner arthritic disorders are mostly non-Mendelian, but some of the major genes involved are becoming apparent, as a result of studies of associations with the HLA system.

Ankylosing Spondylitis

Until the advent of HLA typing this was 'just another multifactorial disorder'. Discovery of the striking association with HLA B27 has revealed this, or some closely linked gene within t1e HLA region, as probably the main genetic determinant. Emery and Lawrence[11] showed a risk of 5 per cent (7 per cent for males and 2 per cent for females) for clinical disease in first-degree relatives of patients with ankylosing spondylitis. Sixteen per cent showed radiological sacro-iliitis. The HLA type of relatives affects their risk considerably (*see* Chapter 3); the chance of a B27 child of a B27 patient developing clinical ankylosing spondylitis is 9 per cent, compared with a risk of less than 1 per cent for offspring without this antigen.

Rheumatoid Arthritis

An association with specific antigens at the HLA D locus is emerging, but the risks of clinical rheumatoid arthritis to relatives are not high; they appear to be doubled for first-degree relatives, though the incidence of radiological abnormalities is considerably higher. The HLA antigen DRW4 is found in rheumatoid arthritis patients with twice the normal frequency, and is six times more common in familial cases, suggesting that this may be the major genetic determinant in the disorder. The occurrence of positive tests for rheumatoid factor is associated with HLA DRW3[12].

Systemic Lupus Erythematosus

This provides an interesting maternal effect, congenital heart block occurring in a proportion of the infants born to an affected mother. No empiric risks for relatives appear to exist for this disorder, or for allied immunological disturbances such as scleroderma. It is likely that they are low (<5 per cent for first-degree relatives), but family studies might well be expected to show a higher frequency of abnormal tests for relevant antibodies.

Osteoarthritis

This occurs with twice the general population prevalence in first-degree relatives. When associated with Heberden's nodes, the risk is higher, probably threefold; the nodes themselves have been thought to show autosomal dominant inheritance with incomplete penetrance in males, but the fact that they occur more frequently in the relatives of rarer male propositi makes polygenic inheritance likely. No HLA association has been shown.

An unusual concentration of osteoarthritis in a family should arouse suspicion of an underlying bone dysplasia. A remarkable family with degenerative hip disease following autosomal dominant inheritance in four generations has been described[13]. *Table* 11.5 summarizes some of the major Mendelian causes of osteoarthritis, based on the review of Harper and Nuki[13].

Table 11.5. Mendelian forms of osteoarthropathy

Interphalangeal osteoarthrosis	Autosomal dominant
Heberden's nodes	Autosomal dominant (*see text*)
Familial digital osteoarthropathy with avascular necrosis	Autosomal dominant
Hereditary arthro-ophthalmopathy (Stickler)	Autosomal dominant
Osteoarthrosis, platyspondyly and beta-2 globulin deficiency	Autosomal recessive (probable)
Multiple epiphyseal dysplasia	Autosomal dominant
Spondylo-epiphyseal dysplasia tarda	X-linked recessive
Pseudoachondroplasia	Autosomal dominant or Autosomal recessive
Hereditary osteoarthritis of the hip	Autosomal dominant
Hereditary chondrocalcinosis	Autosomal dominant or Autosomal recessive
Alkaptonuria	Autosomal recessive

Table 11.6. Recurrence risks for congenital dislocation of the hip (from Wynne-Davies)

Individual affected	*Individual at risk*	*Risk (%)*		
		Overall	♂	♀
One sib	Sibs	6	1	11
One parent	Children	12	6	17
One parent + one child	Children	36		
Second-degree relative	Nephews, nieces	<1		

Congenital Dislocation of the Hip

Apart from environmental factors, it is likely that a genetic contribution is provided both by the shape of the acetabulum and by joint laxity. The sex ratio is about 3 : 1 female to male, and there is marked social class variation. The overall incidence is around 5 per 1000 births. Recurrence risks have been studied by Wynne-Davies[14] whose data are shown in *Table* 11.6. Care must be taken to distinguish transient 'clicking hips' in newborns, and other generalized bone and connective tissue disorders which commonly present with hip dislocation.

Perthes' Disease

True Perthes' disease carries a low recurrence risk, around 0·6 per cent in sibs and 2·8 per cent in children of affected patients[15]. The risks do not appear to be higher in the relatives of patients with bilateral hip disease. Risks for second- and third-degree relatives are minimal. Familial concentrations should arouse suspicion that some other disorder, such as multiple epiphyseal dysplasia, may be present.

Arthrogryposis
A primary diagnosis is essential here; some of the causes are basically neurological, others due to abnormality of skeletal or ligamentous development, while some appear to result from intrauterine restriction.

Major causes in the first group include various congenital myopathies, congenital myotonic dystrophy, and severe spinal muscular atrophy. Skeletal causes are usually confined to specific joints, but a full skeletal survey is important to recognize an underlying bony disorder. One is left with a residue of 'idiopathic' arthrogryposis multiplex congenita in which the ultimate prognosis is good and recurrence in a family is rare. Where two sibs have been affected, even without a specific underlying cause, autosomal recessive inheritance should be suspected.

Talipes
As with arthrogryposis, there are many primary causes, in particular neurological defects, which must be excluded. Idiopathic talipes occurs around 1 in 1000 births in Great Britain, with a male : female ratio of 2 : 1. The risk to sibs is around 3 per cent overall, the risk for sibs of a male patient being lower (2 per cent) than those of a female patient (5 per cent), as expected on the basis of polygenic inheritance. Full data for risks to offspring of patients are not yet available. Wynne-Davies[16] suggests the risk may be as high as 25 per cent for further offspring of an affected parent with an affected child.

There appears to be an increased risk of talipes in children born after amniocentesis (*see* p. 93).

Idiopathic Scoliosis[17]
This may be infantile or adolescent.

Infantile: The incidence is around 1·3 per 1000 births in Great Britain, but much less in N. America. Satisfactory figures for sibs are not available.

Adolescent: The incidence is around 0·3 per 1000 births in boys and 4 per 1000 births in girls. The overall risk for first-degree relatives is around 5−7 per cent for major defects, but data are insufficient to split by sex and type of relative.

Dupuytren's Contracture
When there is no primary cause, the inheritance is thought to be autosomal dominant, but if this is so one might have expected severe forms due to homozygosity for such a common condition.

Hereditary Digital Clubbing

This common and harmless autosomal dominant trait is frequently confused by doctors with acquired clubbing of more serious import. Patients usually correctly recognize its hereditary nature.

Various Skeletal Syndromes

Nail–patella Syndrome (autosomal dominant)

This may present with talipes or hip dislocation in addition to the dysplastic nails and absent patellae. Renal involvement may occur in later life. Linkage with the ABO blood group system could allow prediction in some families, but is unlikely to be of much practical help since the features are usually obvious in early life.

Craniocarpotarsal (Freeman–Sheldon or 'whistling face') syndrome

The hand deformity superficially resembles severe rheumatoid disease, but the lack of X-ray changes and characteristic pinched face should allow recognition of the syndrome. Inheritance is usually autosomal dominant, but affected sibs born to normal consanguineous parents suggests a recessive form also.

Rubinstein–Taybi Syndrome

Broad thumbs and great toes, moderate mental retardation and characteristic facies are the principal features. Recurrence in a family is rare, but patients do not usually reproduce.

Larsen's Syndrome

This combination of multiple dislocations with an unusual facies (and often cleft palate) was originally thought to be autosomal recessive, but parent–child transmission has now been reported so the situation is not clear. Heterogeneity is likely.

Klippel–Feil Syndrome

Many causes of a short neck find their way into this category, but it remains heterogeneous even after their removal. Where the case is an isolated one, the risk for sibs is probably low, though minor degrees of cervical vertebral fusion may be more frequent in relatives. Congenital heart disease is a common accompaniment in patients. Careful clinical assessment and full skeletal survey should allow future delineation of specific entities within this group.

De Lange's Syndrome

Low birth weight dwarfism, mental retardation, characteristic facies with synophrys, and a variety of limb defects are the principal features of this rather unsatisfactory syndrome. Although not obviously heterogeneous, it does not 'hang together' well as a single entity. There is no clear inheritance pattern and no obvious causative factors are known, though a variety of chromosomal defects have been found in a proportion of cases. The risk to sibs is around 2 per cent.

Popliteal Pterygium Syndrome

The multiple pterygia are associated with cleft lip or palate, cryptorchidism, and often syndactyly. Inheritance may be either autosomal dominant or recessive.

Sacral Agenesis

Almost all cases are sporadic, but there seems to be a specific association with maternal diabetes mellitus. There does not appear to be an association with neural tube defects (Chapter 10).

References

1. McKusick V. A., Kelley T. E. and Dorst J. P. (1973) Observations suggesting allelism of the achondroplasia and hypochondroplasia genes. *J. Med. Genet.* **10**, 11–16.
2. Holzgreve W., Carey J. C. and Hall B. D. (1976) Warfarin induced fetal abnormalities. *Lancet* **2**, 914–915.
3. Pena S. D. J. and Goodman H. O. (1973) The genetics of thanatophoric dwarfism. *Pediatrics* **51**, 104–109.
4. David T. J. (1972) Nature and etiology of the Poland anomaly. *N. Engl. J. Med.* **287**, 487–489.
5. Emery A. E. H. (1977) A problem for genetic counselling – split hand deformity. *Clin. Genet.* **12**, 125–127.
6. Luthy D. A., Hall J. G. and Graham C. B. (1979) Prenatal diagnosis of thrombocytopaenia with absent radii. *Clin. Genet.* **15**, 495–499.
7. Sillence D. O., Senn A. and Danks D. M. (1979) Genetic heterogeneity in osteogenesis imperfecta. *J. Med. Genet.* **16**, 101–116.
8. Young I. D. and Harper P. S. (1980) Recurrence risks in osteogenesis imperfecta congenita. *Lancet* **1**, 432.
9. Pope F. M. (1974) Autosomal dominant pseudoxanthoma elasticum. *J. Med. Genet.* **11**, 152–157.
10. Nwokoro N. and Neufeld E. (1979) Detection of Hunter heterozygotes by enzymatic analysis of hair roots. *Am. J. Hum. Genet.* **31**, 42–49.
11. Emery A. E. H. and Lawrence J. S. (1967) Genetics of ankylosing spondylitis. *J. Med. Genet.* **4**, 239–244.
12. Panayi G. S. (1979) Genetic and environmental factors in the pathogenesis of rheumatoid arthritis. In: Harper P. S. and Muir J. (ed.), *Advanced Medicine* **15**, London, Pitman, pp. 96–103.
13. Harper P. S. and Nuki G. (1980) Genetic factors in osteoarthrosis. In: Nuki G. (ed.), *Osteoarthrosis*. London, Pitman.
14. Wynne-Davies R. (1970) A family study of neonatal and late-diagnosis congenital dislocation of the hip. *J. Med. Genet.* **7**, 315.
15. Harper P. S., Brotherton B. J. and Cochlin D. (1976) Genetic risks in Perthes' disease. *Clin. Genet.* **10**, 178–182.
16. Wynne-Davies R. (1965) Family studies and aetiology of clubfoot. *J. Med. Genet.* **2**, 227.
17. Wynne-Davies R. (1968) Familial (idiopathic) scoliosis. *J. Bone Joint Surg.* **50B**, 24–30.

Further Reading

Beighton P. (1978) *Inherited Disorders of the Skeleton.* London, Churchill Livingstone.

McKusick V. A. (1972) *Heritable Disorders of Connective Tissue.* St. Louis, Mosby.

Spranger, J. W., Langer L. O. and Wiedemann H. R. (1974) *Bone Dysplasias. An Atlas of Constitutional Disorders of Skeletal Development.* Philadelphia, Saunders.

Temtamy S. and McKusick V. A. (1978) *The Genetics of Hand Malformations.* New York, Alan Liss.

Wynne-Davies R. (1973) *Heritable Disorders in Orthopaedic Practice.* Oxford, Blackwell.

CHAPTER TWELVE

Oral and Craniofacial Disorders

For most clinicians this is a confusing area, on the borderline between medicine and dentistry, yet overlapping broadly into other fields. The plastic surgeon is the person who sees most of the facial disorders, and there is no doubt that genetic counselling is an integral part of management of these patients; even minor facial anomalies can cause great distress and accurate information regarding possible risks to offspring will provide great relief from worry for such people.

The amount of information available on the inheritance of these disorders is considerable. A surprisingly large number of medical geneticists have begun their careers as dentists and have provided some thorough reviews which are listed at the end of this chapter.

The Teeth

Hypodontia, or lack of one or a few permanent teeth, is extremely common (5–10 per cent in most surveys) and is often inherited as a variable autosomal dominant trait. Complete *anodontia* is usually associated with anhidrotic ectodermal dysplasia (X-linked recessive), but can also occur in the orofaciodigital syndrome (? X-linked dominant).

Enamel defects (amelogenesis imperfecta) provide some well-studied Mendelian disorders including:

Pitted hypoplastic enamel – autosomal dominant (the commonest).

Smooth hypoplastic enamel – autosomal dominant.

X-linked hypoplastic enamel – X-linked dominant.

A combination of the dental features and pedigree pattern should allow the inheritance to be established. General health is normal.

Abnormal enamel may also occur in a number of more general genetic disorders, including familial hypophosphataemic rickets, tuberous sclerosis and several bone dysplasias.

Dentine defects (dentinogenesis imperfecta). The characteristic feature is opalescence or translucency of the teeth. There are two main types:

1. Associated with osteogenesis imperfecta. The dental defect tends to be mild and variable, but may be a useful confirmatory feature in establishing the diagnosis of this variable dominant disease.

2. Isolated dentinogenesis imperfecta. Here the dental defect is much more obvious. Bones are *not* affected. Inheritance is also autosomal dominant.

A number of other types of dentine abnormality also exist, some associated with primary bone disorders.

Cleft Lip and Palate

Before genetic counselling is given, a careful examination must be made to exclude the numerous syndromal associations with clefting. In some of these (e.g. chromosomal trisomies) the other defects are obvious; in others

Table 12.1. Some major syndromes associated with cleft lip and palate

Autosomal dominant
  Lip pits with cleft lip/palate
  EEC syndrome (ectrodactyly, ectodermal dysplasia and clefting)
  Hereditary arthro-ophthalmopathy (Stickler's syndrome)
  Retinal detachment, myopia and cleft palate (Marshall's syndrome)
  Spondylo-epiphyseal dysplasia congenita

Autosomal recessive
  Chondrodysplasia punctata (Conradi's syndrome)
  Larsen's syndrome
  Diastrophic dwarfism
  Smith—Lemli—Opitz syndrome
  Meckel's syndrome
  Orofaciodigital syndrome, type II

X-linked
  Orofaciodigital syndrome, type I
  Otopalatodigital syndrome

Chromosomal
  Trisomy 13
  Trisomy 18
  Chromosome 18 deletions
  Various other autosomal abnormalities

Non-Mendelian
  Pierre Robin syndrome
  Clefting with congenital heart disease
  De Lange's syndrome

(e.g. the lip-pits syndrome) they may be inconspicuous and even absent in some family members. Most important to recognize are those syndromes following Mendelian inheritance. *Table* 12.1 lists some of the major syndromes; fuller lists are given in some excellent reviews listed at the end of the chapter. Cleft lip and palate also occur with other malformations in a non-specific manner more commonly than expected. If a careful search for a 'specific' syndrome proves negative, one is forced to use the empiric risks for the abnormalities in isolation. The possibility of fetoscopy should be considered in a serious clefting syndrome with a high recurrence risk.

Numerous studies have shown that cleft palate alone runs separately in families from cleft lip with or without cleft palate. *Table* 12.2 summarizes the overall risks based on a number of primary European and American sources[1, 2, 3, 4]. There is little difference in risk to males or females, but as expected with polygenic inheritance the presence of other affected family members considerably raises the risks. The population incidence of cleft lip (with or without cleft palate) is 1 in 500 to 1 in 1000, compared with around 1 in 2500 for isolated cleft palate. One point to note from *Table* 12.2 is that the risk for sibs of a patient with cleft lip/palate is less

Table 12.2 Cleft lip and palate – genetic risks[1, 2, 3, 4]

Relationship to index case	Cleft lip ± palate	Isolated cleft palate
Sibs (overall risk)	4·0%	1·8%
Sib (no other affected members)	2·2%	
Sib (2 affected sibs)	10%	8%
Sib + affected parent	10%	
Children	4·3%	6·2%
Second-degree relatives	0·6%	
Third-degree relatives	0·3%	
General population	0·1%	0·04%

Table 12.3. Genetic risks in cleft lip/palate: effect of severity

	Risk to sibs (%)
Bilateral cleft lip + palate	5·7
Unilateral cleft lip + palate	4·2
Unilateral cleft lip alone	2·5

when it can be definitely established that no other relatives are affected (2·2 per cent) than is the overall risk to sibs (4 per cent) found by surveys, which will include some families with other affected relatives of varying closeness. Therefore, this higher risk should be used when family information is unavailable or unreliable. Some data are now available on the influence of severity (*Table* 12.3) and as expected there is a higher risk when the abnormality is bilateral and a lower risk when there is only cleft lip.

Pierre Robin Syndrome (Cleft palate with mandibular hypoplasia)
Mandibular hypoplasia, with or without cleft palate and with resulting respiratory obstruction from the tongue, may be part of a variety of

skeletal or muscular syndromes, some Mendelian (e.g. congenital myotonic dystrophy). In the absence of these, the risk of recurrence is low; the prognosis for patients with careful treatment is good.

Aphthous Ulcers of the Mouth
Around 20–25 per cent of the general population suffer from this minor, but tiresome complaint to some degree, and around 40 per cent of first-degree relatives appear to be affected.

Gingival Fibromatosis
Though most commonly seen as a result of phenytoin treatment, this may occur as an isolated autosomal dominant trait, as well as in some more general syndromes.

Aglossia–adactylia
Recurrence in sibs has not been noted, but insufficient patients have reproduced to exclude new dominant mutation as the cause.

Atrophic Rhinitis
Although most cases are sporadic, occasional families following a clear autosomal dominant pattern have been documented.

Craniofacial Syndromes
Acrocephalosyndactyly
Several specific genetic and clinical types exist, which it is important to distinguish in genetic counselling.

1. Apert's syndrome (severe cranial stenosis, fusion of most digits, frequent mental retardation). Autosomal dominant with most patients new mutations.

2. Chotzen's syndrome (milder cranial stenosis; digital fusion mostly soft tissue and of digits 2–4). Autosomal dominant.

3. Pfeiffer type (mild acrocephaly with broad thumbs and great toes and partial digital fusion). Autosomal dominant.

4. Summitt type (mild acrocephaly and digital fusion with hypogonadism and obesity. Probably autosomal recessive.

5. Acrocephalopolysyndactyly (Carpenter's syndrome). Autosomal recessive. Frequently severe; fetoscopy may prove helpful.

Crouzon's Disease (Craniofacial dysostosis)
Involvement of the orbits and midface as well as the cranium, gives a characteristic appearance. Inheritance is autosomal dominant.

Isolated Craniostenosis
Most cases are sporadic, regardless of which sutures are involved; recurrence risks are low, but not well defined. Occasional families with clear

autosomal recessive inheritance have been described, so if multiple family members are affected it is wise to assume that one is dealing with a Mendelian type.

Mandibulofacial Dysostosis (Treacher Collins syndrome)
Severity of the facial abnormality varies greatly but inheritance is autosomal dominant. Deafness is a common feature in addition to external ear defects; mental retardation is said to occur, but is possibly an artefact of ascertainment. Potential parents will tend to be milder than average and must be warned that an affected child could be considerably more affected. A separate syndrome of mandibulofacial dysostosis with preaxial limb defects follows autosomal recessive inheritance.

Hallermann–Streiff Syndrome (Oculomandibulofacial syndrome; François' dyscephalic syndrome)
Congenital cataracts, short stature, beaked nose with micrognathia and characteristic facies are all features of this disorder. Inheritance is probably autosomal dominant with most patients new mutations, but few patients have reproduced. The risk of recurrence in sibs is minimal.

Goldenhar's Syndrome (Oculo-auriculovertebral dysplasia)
This must be distinguished from the superficially similar Treacher Collins syndrome. The external ear defects are more marked, mental retardation is usual and epibulbar dermoid cyst of the eye is characteristic. Most cases are sporadic, and the recurrence risk where parents are normal is low.

Hemifacial Microsomia
Unilateral hypoplasia of most facial structures is the characteristic feature. Recurrence is exceptional.

Sturge–Weber Syndrome
This must be distinguished from other angiomatous malformations of the face. The involvement of the ophthalmic trigeminal area and extension to deep tissues of skull and meninges are characteristic, as is congenital glaucoma. No causative factors are known, but the condition is almost always sporadic.

Orofaciodigital Syndrome
Characteristic features are clefting of jaw and tongue, with digital abnormalities (usually syndactyly) and sometimes mental retardation. Almost all cases are female, suggesting X-linked dominant inheritance lethal in the male (*see* Chapter 2). A risk of 50 per cent for female offspring should be given. An extremely rare form (type II) following autosomal recessive inheritance and clinically distinguishable, has been described.

Frontonasal Dysplasia and Median Cleft Face Syndrome

Almost all cases have been sporadic, but affected individuals rarely reproduce.

Aarskog's Syndrome

This X-linked recessive disorder combines hypertelorism with digital and spinal abnormalities and characteristic scrotal shape.

References

1. Fogh-Andersen P. (1942) *Inheritance of Hare Lip and Cleft Palate.* Copenhagen, Munksgaard.
2. Bixler D., Fogh-Andersen P. and Conneally P. M. (1971) Incidence of cleft lip and palate in the offspring of cleft parents. *Clin. Genet.* **2,** 155–159.
3. Woolf C. M. (1971) Congenital cleft lip. A genetic study of 496 propositi. *J. Med. Genet.* **8,** 65–71.
4. Shapiro B. L. (1976) The genetics of cleft lip and palate. In: Stewart R. E. and Prescott G. H. (ed.), *Oral Facial Genetics.* St Louis, Mosby. pp. 473–499.

Further Reading

Bergsma D. (ed.) (1971) *The Clinical Delineation of Birth Defects,* Part XI. *Orofacial Structures.* Baltimore, Wilkins & Wilkins.
Goodman R. M. and Gorlin R. J. (1977) *Atlas of the Face in Genetic Disorders.* St Louis, Mosby.
Gorlin R. J. and Pindborg J. J. (1964) *Syndromes of the Head and Neck.* New York, McGraw-Hill.
Stewart R. E. and Prescott G. H. (ed.) (1976) *Oral Facial Genetics.* St Louis, Mosby. (The chapter, Dysmorphic Syndromes with Craniofacial Manifestations, by M. M. Cohen, ranks almost as a separate work in its own right.)

CHAPTER THIRTEEN

The Skin

A high proportion of disorders affecting the skin and its appendages follow Mendelian inheritance, and because they are readily available for inspection, are easier than most to document in families. Since skin disorders are rarely fatal and interfere relatively little with reproduction it is often possible to identify with confidence what mode of inheritance is operating, even if one is rather ignorant of the precise pathology or aetiology of the condition. It must be remembered, however, that skin lesions may be the external marker for more serious internal or generalized disease, and that even their cosmetic effect may be considered much more serious by the patient than the physician.

Most of the Mendelian disorders in this chapter are simply tabulated, without an attempt to describe them (*Table* 13.1). Useful sources are given at the end of the chapter.

Table 13.1. Skin disorders following Mendelian inheritance

Autosomal dominant
    Acanthosis nigricans
    Acrokeratosis verruciformis
    Angioneurotic oedema
    Basal-cell naevus syndrome
    Blue rubber bleb naevus
    Cutis laxa (also autosomal recessive)
    Cylindromatosis (turban tumours)
    Ectodermal dysplasia, hidrotic type and EEC syndrome
    Epidermolysis bullosa, simplex and Cockayne types, and most dystrophic cases
    Epithelioma, multiple self-healing
    Erythrokeratodermia variabilis
    Glomus tumours, multiple
    Hailey–Hailey disease (benign familial pemphigus)
    Ichthyosis hystrix
    Ichthyosis vulgaris
    Keratosis follicularis (Darier's disease); most families
    Koilonychia, hereditary
    Mastocytosis, familial
    Monilethrix
    Nail–patella syndrome
    Neurofibromatosis

    Palmo-plantar hyperkeratosis (tylosis)
    Porokeratosis of Mibelli
    Porphyria (all types except congenital erythropoietic)
    Porphyria variegata
    Steatocystoma multiplex
    Hereditary haemorrhagic telangiectasia
    Tuberous sclerosis

Autosomal recessive
    Acrodermatitis enteropathica
    Albinism, oculocutaneous
    Ataxia telangiectasia
    Bloom's syndrome
    Chediak—Higashi syndrome
    Chondro-ectodermal dysplasia (Ellis—van Creveld)
    Cockayne's syndrome
    Cutis laxa (also autosomal dominant)
    Epidermolysis bullosa (letalis and some dystrophic forms)
    Ichthyosis, congenita and other types (*see* p. 182)
    Lipoid proteinosis
    Netherton's syndrome
    Palmo-plantar hyperkeratosis (Mal de Meleda and Papillon—Lefèvre
       types)
    Pili torti
    Porphyria, congenital erythropoietic
    Progeria
    Pseudoxanthoma elasticum
    Rothmund—Thompson syndrome
    Seip's lipodystrophy syndrome
    Werner's syndrome
    Xeroderma pigmentosum

X-linked (recessive unless stated)
    Dyskeratosis congenita
    Ectodermal dysplasia, anhidrotic
    Fabry's disease
    Focal dermal hypoplasia (? dominant, lethal in male)
    Chronic granulomatous disease
    Ichthyosis, X-linked
    Incontinentia pigmenti (? dominant, lethal in male)
    Keratosis follicularis spinulosa (dominant)
    Menkes 'kinky hair' syndrome
    Wiskott—Aldrich syndrome

Skin Colour

Inheritance is polygenic, with probably 5 or 6 genes of additive effect at several loci. Advice is frequently sought regarding the offspring of inter-racial marriages or adoptions, and questions on this subject may merely be the focusing point of a considerable amount of stress, ignorance and latent prejudice. The attitude of other family members such as in-laws or grand-parents may be frankly hostile, and it may in fact often be not so much skin colour as other racial characteristics, such as hair or facial features, that are the main concern.

In general, any children will be likely to show skin colour intermediate between that of the parents; where both parents are of mixed race this will still apply, but here the likelihood is greater that a child may be either darker or lighter than both parents as a result of inheriting a particular selection of pigment-determining genes.

Light-skinned individuals of mixed race married to a white person may enquire whether a child or subsequent descendant might have extremely dark skin colour or African features; in other words, that he might be a clearly Black person who might not be accepted in the White community into which he has been born. This is very unlikely, but again it cannot be excluded that the degree of pigmentation, though probably not of other features, might exceed that of the darker parent, especially if the 'white' partner is relatively dark skinned. Where he or she is blond and light-skinned, this possibility can be discounted.

Where mixed race origin is known or is a possibility, caution must be advised in predicting later appearance from features present in early infancy. Skin colour may darken significantly and African-origin hair may not be apparent for some months after birth. Reed[1] writing in 1955, deals in detail with these various features and it is of interest that inheritance of skin colour was the commonest reason for seeking genetic counselling at his clinic. Although the climate of opinion has significantly altered since that time, and inter-racial marriages and adoptions are now more frequent and accepted, one should not underestimate the significance to families of what might, to the physician, appear trivial features.

When adoption is being considered the essential point is that the adoptive parents should know what to expect and should accept the situation; if they do not, the later problems for both child and parents can indeed be serious.

Psoriasis[2]

This common and variable disorder (prevalence around 1–2 per cent) is frequently familial. Families apparently following all major types of Mendelian inheritance have been reported, but it is likely that most of these represent extreme examples of a disorder that is polygenically determined. An association has been found with the HLA antigen CW6.

The risk for first-degree relatives of an isolated case is at least 10 per cent, and probably double this where there are two affected first-degree relatives. Where the disorder appears to follow an autosomal dominant pattern, it is probably wise to give a risk approaching 50 per cent for offspring of an affected member, but it is doubtful whether unaffected members of such pedigrees are completely free from the risk of transmitting it.

The children of two psoriatic patients also have a risk of around 50 per cent of being affected, but there does not seem to be a specially severe form in such children, as might be expected if homozygosity at a single gene locus were operating.

Atopic Eczema

This extremely common problem, often associated with asthma and other allergic phenomena, is probably determined by an autosomal dominant gene of rather variable expression, though we do not yet have a reliable immunological marker for its presence. The risk of some allergic problem where one parent is affected approaches 50 per cent, and is somewhat higher where both parents are affected, though it does not appear that homozygosity results in a particularly severe clinical picture.

The Ichthyoses (*Table* 13.2)

It is usually possible to distinguish different types on clinical and histological grounds as well as genetically, so that with care correct counselling can be given even for isolated cases. Thus severe ichthyosis in a neonate

Table 13.2. The inherited ichthyoses[13]

Disorder	Inheritance
Ichthyosis without syndromal association	
Congenital ichthyosis	
a. Lamellar ichthyosis (collodion baby)	Autosomal recessive
b. Harlequin fetus (lethal)	Autosomal recessive
Ichthyosis hystrix	Autosomal dominant
Ichthyosis vulgaris	Autosomal dominant
X-linked ichthyosis	X-linked recessive
Syndromes associated with ichthyosis	
Refsum's syndrome	Autosomal recessive
Ichthyosis with mental retardation and spastic tetraplegia	
(Sjögren—Larsson syndrome)	Autosomal recessive
Ichthyosis with male hypogonadism	X-linked recessive
Conradi's syndrome (chondrodysplasia punctata)	Autosomal dominant or autosomal recessive
Ichthyosiform erythroderma with deafness	Autosomal recessive
Ichthyosiform erythroderma with unilateral limb defects	Autosomal recessive
Ichthyosis congenita with cataract	Autosomal recessive
Ichthyosis with mental retardation and hypogonadism	
(Rud's syndrome)	Autosomal recessive

almost certainly follows autosomal recessive inheritance, while mild ichthyosis in a female is likely to be autosomal dominant. A deficiency of steroid sulphatase has recently been shown to be responsible for X-linked ichthyosis[3] and should prove of diagnostic help. A careful general examination to exclude the various generalized syndromes is important.

Palmo-plantar Hyperkeratosis (tylosis)

Most cases follow autosomal dominant inheritance and isolated cases thus have a high risk of transmitting the disorder. The rare form known as 'Mal de Meleda' is autosomal recessive and does occur in Britain. The remarkable families with dominantly inherited oesophageal cancer and tylosis[4] have late childhood onset of the skin disorder. They are exceptional and families with tylosis from early childhood, but no history of oesophageal cancer in the family, should not be worried by this possibility being mentioned.

Epidermolysis Bullosa[5]

This is another heterogeneous group in which genetic differences are supported by the clinical and histological features. Thus the neonatal 'letalis' form (now treatable by steroids) is autosomal recessive, while the mild 'simplex' types, without scarring, are autosomal dominant. The dystrophic forms with scarring may follow either pattern, but most severe cases are autosomal recessive.

Prenatal diagnosis of the 'letalis' form by fetoscopic skin biopsy has recently been reported[6].

Ectodermal Dysplasias

Anhidrotic ectodermal dysplasia. The commonest disorder in this group is X-linked recessive, with variable expression in female carriers, who may show dental anomalies as well as a reduced sweat pore count. Unfortunately, complete normality does not exclude the carrier state and in one personally studied case a completely normal mother later had a second affected son. For an isolated case, it is probably wise to assume a risk of at least two-thirds that the mother is a carrier with a corresponding risk of one-third for her daughters. It is not known to what degree absence of clinical abnormalities reduces these risks. A worrying feature in counselling is the occurrence of mental retardation in some cases; it is uncertain whether this is always secondary to hyperpyrexia. Other types of ectodermal dysplasia are autosomal; both dominant and recessive types have been described, as well as a number of syndromes (*see* EEC syndrome, p. 163 and chondro-ectodermal dysplasia, p. 162.

Naevi

Pigmented naevi in a particular site commonly follow autosomal dominant inheritance. Multiple pigmented naevi are a feature of Turner's syndrome and of the dominantly inherited syndrome of multiple naevi with nerve deafness (leopard syndrome). The skin lesions of neurofibromatosis and tuberous sclerosis must be distinguished, as must lesions overlying a spina bifida.

Cavernous haemangiomas of the facial region are usually sporadic, as is the trigeminal area flat vascular naevus of the *Sturge–Weber syndrome.*

Haemangiomatous and lymphangiomatous lesions of the limbs may be associated with hypertrophy and are also usually sporadic, though familial cases are described (*see* Chapter 22); rare instances of autosomal dominant inheritance in association with Wilms tumour have also been recorded. Other specific types of naevus following autosomal dominant inheritance are naevus flammeus of the nape of the neck, the 'blue rubber bleb' multiple naevi, and multiple glomus tumours.

Albinism
Generalized oculocutaneous albinism is autosomal recessive. Two main types exist: a severe form (tyrosinase-negative) with total lack of pigment throughout life, and a milder (tyrosinase-positive) form in which pigmentation of hair and iris gradually increases and in which mild cases may easily be missed. The forms are non-allelic, since marriages between albinos of different type result in all normal offspring, whereas when both are of the same type all are affected [7]. Children of albinos married to non-albinos will, of course generally be normal, though heterozygotes are often detectable by translucency of the iris. A very rare type, associated with a bleeding diathesis (Hermansky–Pudlak syndrome) is also autosomal recessive.

Ocular albinism (*see* Chapter 14) is X-linked.

Vitiligo
This is commonly associated with a variety of autoimmune endocrine disturbances and like them often follows a variable autosomal dominant pattern.

Piebaldism
Isolated white forelock may occur as a dominantly inherited trait, but may be part of the more generalized Waardenburg syndrome (p. 200) also autosomal dominant in inheritance.

Baldness
Severe, early male baldness is probably due to autosomal dominant inheritance, with expression of the gene limited to the male unless it is present in homozygous state. Premature balding is a feature of myotonic dystrophy. Hair loss or sparsity may also result from a variety of ectodermal dysplasias and specific hair disorders (e.g. monilethrix, pili torti). Alopoecia areata is often associated with autoimmune endocrine disorders.

Acanthosis Nigricans
Primary acanthosis nigricans starts early in life and follows autosomal dominant inheritance. Acanthosis nigricans may also accompany a variety of other genetic disorders; onset in later life is commonly an indication of acquired visceral malignancy. The inherited type has no such association.

Skin Tumours

A remarkable number of the rarer skin or skin-related tumours follow Mendelian inheritance, mostly autosomal dominant, and appear in the lists in *Table* 13.1 and *Table* 22.1, p. 246. The recessively inherited disorders of DNA repair also frequently present with skin manifestations.

Xeroderma Pigmentosum

This disorder (autosomal recessive) is now detectable prenatally[8] as a repair defect of U-V induced DNA damage. Since several separate types exist[9] it is important for the cultured cells of the affected sib to be studied before embarking on prenatal diagnosis.

Kaposi's Sarcoma

Most cases are sporadic and there is marked geographical variation in incidence, probably not genetic in origin. Risks to family members are low except in the small, but well documented number of families with multiple cases[10].

Malignant Melanoma

Most cases appear to be non-genetic, but autosomal dominant inheritance occurs in a few striking families[11]. Transplacental passage of malignant cells is also recorded.

Basal-cell Naevus Syndrome[12]

This dominantly inherited disorder may be recognizable from skeletal abnormalities, especially jaw cysts, before skin tumours appear. There may be an increased risk of cerebral tumours also. Isolated basal-cell tumours are not known to be genetic.

Epitheliomas

No definite genetic tendency is known except for the rare and remarkable familial *self-healing epithelioma* known principally from Western Scotland.

Congenital Fibromatosis

In this rare disorder, multiple spindle-cell fibromatous tumours occur and commonly mature spontaneously. The condition may be fatal if gut tumours occur but is usually benign. Although autosomal recessive inheritance has been claimed, autosomal dominant inheritance with incomplete penetrance (especially in older individuals) is more probable. Careful search for small lesions in apparently unaffected parents is important.

References
1. Reed S. C. (1955) *Counselling in Medical Genetics.* Philadelphia, Saunders.
2. Watson W., Cann H. M., Farber E. M. et al. (1972) The genetics of psoriasis. *Arch. Derm.* **105,** 197–207.

3. Shapiro L. J., Weiss R., Webster D. and France J. T. (1978) X-linked ichthyosis due to steroid-sulphatase deficiency. *Lancet* 1, 70–72.
4. Harper P. S., Harper R. M. J. and Howel-Evans A. W. (1970) Carcinoma of the oesophagus with tylosis. *Q. J. Med.* 39, 317–333.
5. Gedde-Dahl T. (1971) *Epidermolysis Bullosa. A Clinical, Genetic and Epidemiological Study.* Baltimore, Johns Hopkins University Press.
6. Rodeck C. H., Eady R. A. J. and Gosden C. M. (1980) Prenatal diagnosis of epidermolysis bullosa letalis. *Lancet* 1, 949–952.
7. Trevor-Roper P. D. (1963) Marriage of two complete albinos with normally pigmented offspring. *Proc. R. Soc. Med.* 56, 21–24.
8. Regan J. D., Setlow R. B., Kaback M. M. et al. (1971) Xeroderma pigmentosum: a rapid sensitive method for prenatal diagnosis. *Science* 174, 147–150.
9. Robbins J. H., Kraemer K. H., Lutzer M. A. et al. (1974) Xeroderma pigmentosum. An inherited disease with sun sensitivity, multiple cutaneous neoplasms, and abnormal DNA repair. *Ann. Intern. Med.* 80, 221–248.
10. Finlay A. Y. and Marks R. (1979) Familial Kaposi's sarcoma. *Br. J. Dermatol.* 100, 323–326.
11. Anderson D. E. (1971) Clinical characteristics of the genetic variety of cutaneous melanoma in man. *Cancer* 28, 721–725.
12. Gorlin R. J. and Sedano H. O. (1971) The multiple basal cell carcinoma syndrome revisited. In: Bergsma D. (ed.), *The Clinical Delineation of Birth Defects.* 12, p. 140–148. Baltimore, Williams & Wilkins.
13. Harper P. S. (1978) Genetic heterogeneity in the ichthyoses. In: Mark R. and Dykes P. J. (ed.), *The Ichthyoses.* Lancaster, MTP. pp. 127–136.

Further Reading

Bergsma D. (ed.) (1972) *The Clinical Delineation of Birth Defects.* 12, Skin, hair and nails. Baltimore, Williams & Wilkins.
Kaloustian V. M. Der and Hurtan A. K. (1979) *Genetic Disease of the Skin.* Berlin, Springer.
Marks R. and Dykes P. J. (ed.) (1978) *The Ichthyoses.* Lancaster, MTP.

CHAPTER FOURTEEN

The Eye

Not only are many of the major eye disorders largely genetic in origin, but they have been exceptionally thoroughly documented from the genetic as well as the clinical viewpoint. Many of the pioneers in clinical genetics have been ophthalmologists, and a number of encyclopaedic works exist

Table 14.1. X-linked eye disorders

Disorder	Changes in heterozygote
Ocular albinism	Patchy fundal depigmentation, translucency of iris
Oculocutaneous albinism with deafness	Partial hearing loss
X-linked congenital cataract	Sutural lens opacities
Choroideraemia	Retinal pigmentary changes (sometimes symptomatic) Abnormal electroretinogram
Colour blindness, deutan	
Colour blindness, protan	
Colour blindness, incomplete achromatopsia	
Iris hypoplasia with glaucoma	
X-linked macular dystrophy	
Megalocornea (also rarely autosomal dominant)	
Microphthalmos with multiple anomalies (Lenz syndrome)	
Congenital night blindness with myopia	
Norrie's disease (pseudoglioma)	
Hereditary nystagmus	Variable; may be fully affected
Oculocerebrorenal (Lowe) syndrome	Mild lens opacities
X-linked retinitis pigmentosa	Patchy retinal pigmentary and electroretinographic changes
Retinoschisis	
Fabry's disease	Corneal and lens opacities

on ophthalmic genetics which give a wealth of detail. Despite this admirable foundation, however, it has to be said that many ophthalmologists do not give genetic counselling a high priority, and that many patients and relatives, including those with severe visual loss, receive no advice on the genetic risks until after they have had their families. This is particularly sad in an area which offers such scope for prevention.

Patients with congenital or childhood blindness frequently marry each other, with complex results, though in contrast to congenital deafness it is usually possible to distinguish the precise genetic type of each parent's disorder. The author has found a clinic at a school for the visually handicapped, run jointly with an ophthalmologist, of great help to school leavers and their parents. Such schools serve a wide geographical area and allow many patients to be seen who might have been missed through the regular genetic advisory service. Such a system also minimizes the risk of erroneous diagnosis, which a non-specialist is in no position to query by himself.

Since this chapter cannot possibly list, let alone discuss all the hereditary ophthalmic disorders, a selective approach has been adopted, aimed to help the paediatricians and other non-ophthalmic clinicians who encounter hereditary eye disorders. It is *not* intended for ophthalmologists, though they may perhaps find some parts helpful.

A remarkable number of X-linked disorders affecting the eye are known, and these are listed in full (*Table* 14.1) since they produce special problems in counselling. The carrier state can be recognized in a number of these and they provide direct evidence for mosaicism due to X chromosome inactivation in the female. Patchy morphological changes can be seen in a number of these carriers which allow diagnosis of the carrier state in the absence of biochemical tests.

Choroidoretinal Degenerations

A great variety of types exists, characterized by particular features of fundal appearance, by differences in severity and progression, and by different responses to various types of investigation. It is most unwise for the non-ophthalmologist to venture into diagnosis here, but he can make a valuable contribution by documenting the pedigree pattern and by carefully searching for any associated syndromic features. This information can then be combined with a specific ophthalmic diagnosis to allow accurate counselling. An idea of the complexity of the field can be seen in the book by Krill (1977). Only a few types are mentioned here.

Retinitis Pigmentosa

This group, the commonest of the retinal degenerations, may follow all three main modes of Mendelian inheritance, autosomal recessive forms being commonest (about a half), with autosomal dominant inheritance accounting for around 15 per cent of families and 5 per cent being X-linked. Marked variation in course occurs in different families, suggesting further heterogeneity. Carriers of the X-linked form usually show visible pigmentary disturbance and abnormal electroretinogram, a useful distinguishing point from the other forms of inheritance in an isolated male case. The carriers for autosomal recessive forms do not generally show abnormalities, so distinction between a new autosomal dominant mutation and an isolated case due to autosomal recessive inheritance is often impossible; clinical features are too variable to help much. The empiric risk for an affected child being born to such an isolated case is around 1 in 8. Should a child indeed be affected, the risk to subsequent offspring would, of course, be 1 in 2.

A number of syndromes with retinitis pigmentosa exist, including the Bardet–Biedl syndrome (with polydactyly, hypogonadism and mental retardation) the Hallgren syndrome (with deafness, ataxia and mental disturbance) and the Usher syndrome (with profound nerve deafness), all being autosomal recessive.

Leber's Congenital Amaurosis (not to be confused with Leber's optic atrophy)
This primary retinal disorder is one of the commonest causes of childhood blindness, and is autosomal recessive in inheritance. The condition can be detected in early infancy by electroretinogram. Occasional families with associated cerebral and renal degeneration are known.

Night Blindness
This is usually autosomal dominant when occurring as an isolated, static disorder. An X-linked recessive form with myopia also exists.

Table 14.2. Hereditary nystagmus in childhood

Cause	Inheritance
Ocular albinism	X-linked recessive
Idiopathic pendular or jerky nystagmus	X-linked dominant (variable in female)
Macular hypoplasia Congenital cone dysfunction Leber's congenital amaurosis Congenital optic atrophy	Autosomal recessive

Nystagmus
A clear primary diagnosis is essential, since the causes may be neurological or vestibular in addition to ocular. Even when the nystagmus is primary, there are a number of causes (*Table* 14.2). Probably the most important to recognize are the various types of albinism and the X-linked 'hereditary jerky nystagmus' which shows very variable manifestation in females (*see Fig.* 2.19, p. 40).

Colour Vision
The common forms of colour blindness, whether protan or deutan in type, are uniformly X-linked recessive in inheritance and occur in about 8 per

cent of males. Because of this high frequency, matings of affected male and carrier female are not uncommon, with a 50 per cent risk of children of either sex being affected. Around 0·4 per cent of women have colour blindness.

The rare total colour blindness (monochromatism) is autosomal recessive in inheritance, apart from the even rarer 'blue cone' type which is X-linked.

Leber's Optic Atrophy (not to be confused with Leber's congenital amaurosis)

This remarkable disorder has puzzled geneticists for many years, and breaks all the rules of Mendelian inheritance! The main genetic features are:

1. Males are affected more often than females (85 per cent).

2. Males *never* transmit the disease to descendants of either sex, not even to grandchildren or subsequent generations.

3. Where a female is affected or has an affected son, the risk to subsequent sons is 1 in 2, but *all* her daughters appear to be either carriers or affected (unlike X-linkage).

Numerous explanations for this unique pattern have been proposed, none of them satisfactory. It seems likely that a maternally transmitted environmental agent (viral?) is involved, with genetic factors (Mendelian?) determining susceptibility.

Corneal Dystrophies

Numerous types exist; the slit-lamp appearance is often very characteristic (to the expert) and unless a clear pedigree pattern exists, it is wise to be guided by ophthalmological opinion. Most types are Mendelian. Corneal clouding and opacification may be a helpful diagnostic feature in various generalized diseases, notably the mucopolysaccharidoses.

This is perhaps an appropriate point to note that the slit-lamp is a most valuable tool in the early diagnosis and carrier detection of many genetic disorders and one that should be used much more widely than it is. The clinical geneticist prepared to learn the use of this instrument will find it a valuable skill; alternatively, a close working relationship with an ophthalmologist colleague should be developed to allow the examination to be done at short notice.

Retinal Detachment

This is commonly associated with high myopia, and a significant risk to relatives is only likely when severe myopia is present in them also. Several other genetic syndromes may be accompanied by retinal detachment, including the Stickler syndrome; the X-linked disorder retinoschisis can be looked on as a special type of retinal detachment.

Retinoblastoma

This provides an extremely important and difficult area for genetic counselling. All bilateral cases appear to be genetic, but only about 15 per cent of unilateral cases. Although it has been suggested that histological distinction of the genetic form is possible, this has not been confirmed, and early irradiation now frequently avoids surgery, so that histology is not available.

Table 14.3. Genetic risks to offspring in unilateral retinoblastoma (after Fuhrmann and Vogel, 1976; *see* Chapter 1 for reference)

	Risk
Affected with affected parent or sib	40%
Unaffected. Parent and sib or 2 sibs affected	6·6%
Affected. No other affected relatives	6%
Unaffected. One affected child	1·6%
Unaffected. One affected sib	<1%

Table 14.4 Genetic risks in bilateral retinoblastoma

	Risk
Affected. Other family members affected	40%
Affected. No other affected family members	40%
Unaffected. One affected child	8%
Unaffected. Parent affected	6·7%

A further problem arises from lack of penetrance; only 80 per cent of those with the gene develop tumours and it is distinctly possible that other unorthodox mechanisms are responsible for the well-documented instances when the action of the gene appears to be suppressed in an entire branch of a kindred. Occasionally, spontaneous disappearance of a tumour may leave a retinal scar as the only feature. Survivors may have an increased risk of other neoplasms in later life.

Most cases of retinoblastoma are not associated with other malformations, but abnormalities of chromosome 13 may be accompanied by retinoblastoma, leading to suggestions that the gene is located on this chromosome.

Leaving aside theoretical problems, the risk of retinoblastoma in various situations is summarized in *Tables* 14.3, 14.4. An extremely clear account is given by Fuhrmann and Vogel (1976), and the risks given in *Tables* 14.3, 14.4 are based on this.

Norrie's Disease (Pseudoglioma)
In the past this disorder was frequently confused with retinoblastoma; the frequent occurrence of mental retardation makes genetic counselling of this X-linked recessive disease of extreme importance. Unfortunately, no methods of carrier detection or of prenatal diagnosis exist.

Cataract
Congenital Cataract
Numerous types exist, with all forms of inheritance recorded. The incidence is around 1 in 250 births. Environmental causes (e.g. rubella) and other primary disorders (e.g. galactosaemia and hypoparathyroidism) must be excluded, and syndromal associations (e.g. Conradi's disease) looked for.

Since most genetic forms without a metabolic cause follow dominant inheritance, the risk for offspring of an affected person is not far short of 50 per cent. The risks for sibs of an isolated case is probably around 1 in 8, but more accurate figures are needed.

Cataracts in Later Life
Primary disorders, both Mendelian (e.g. myotonic dystrophy) and non-Mendelian (e.g. diabetes) must be excluded. Most families showing a clear-cut aggregation appear to follow autosomal dominant inheritance.

Lens Dislocation
This is a feature of the Marfan and Marchesani syndromes and homo-cystinuria, but may occur as an isolated abnormality due to an abnormally small and spherical lens (spherophakia), usually following autosomal dominant inheritance. The author has seen tall and thin members of one such family persistently misdiagnosed as the Marfan syndrome, with much unnecessary worry caused.

Glaucoma
Primary open angle glaucoma is common in the general population and is found in about 1 in 200 elderly people. Studies of sibs have shown between 5 and 16 per cent to be affected; 10 per cent is probably an appropriate risk for clinically significant glaucoma. The risks for children have been lower, but extremely variable. Since the children studied were always much younger than the sibs, it seems likely that the lifetime risk will approach the 10 per cent seen for sibs. The precise mode of inheritance is

arguable. The intra-ocular pressure response to corticosteroids, which appears to be controlled by a single pair of alleles, may be helpful in predicting high risk family members.

Primary closed angle glaucoma seems to be determined largely by anatomical orbital factors, particularly shallowness of the anterior chamber; 12 per cent of sibs were found to be clinically affected in one study.

Congenital glaucoma may be associated with other generalized ocular problems (e.g. retinoblastoma, Sturge—Weber syndrome). When primary a proportion of families appears to follow autosomal recessive inheritance, but isolated cases are much too common for this mode to explain all cases. The risk to sibs after a single affected child is around 10 per cent; after two affected sibs a 25 per cent risk is wise. Risks to children of affected individuals are uncertain. Assuming a mixture of recessive and polygenic forms a risk of 5 per cent seems appropriate until data are available.

Refractive Errors
Twin studies show a very close concordance between monozygotic twin pairs, suggesting a high degree of genetic determinance. Individual pedigrees showing all types of Mendelian inheritance have been produced for each of the major types of refractive error, but are of little help in deriving general risks for relatives. Studies of unselected families show high correlations for refractive values between both sibs and parents and offspring, suggesting that a polygenic basis is present with genes of additive effect and little dominance or recessivity. The same situation applies to disorders of corneal shape such as astigmatism, keratoconus and cornea plana.

Some regular syndromes of refractive error exist, e.g. myopia and night blindness which is usually X-linked recessive. Refractive errors may also accompany other primary Mendelian disorders, e.g. myopia in the Marfan syndrome.

Cyclops
Almost all cases of this lethal malformation have been sporadic; chromosomal abnormalities have been found in some cases.

Microphthalmos and Anophthalmos
This is an extremely heterogeneous group. Unilateral cases are frequently non-genetic, but cannot be securely distinguished from genetic forms. Rubella and toxoplasma are causes to be excluded for bilateral disease. Mental retardation is frequently associated, and microphthalmos is a feature of severe chromosomal defects as well as Mendelian syndromes. The X-linked Lenz syndrome of microphthalmos with cataract, mental retardation, digital and genito-urinary abnormalities must be considered. Microphthalmos with coloboma is usually autosomal dominant (in the absence of known external causes). Complete bilateral anophthalmos is

generally autosomal recessive. Cryptophthalmos, with absent palpebral fissures, may be part of the above disorders, or may occur with relatively normal eye development, usually following autosomal recessive inheritance.

Coloboma and Aniridia
Both isolated bilateral coloboma of the iris and the more severe aniridia usually follow autosomal dominant inheritance; colobomas may form part of more extensive ocular disorders. The rare syndrome of ocular coloboma with anal atresia follows an autosomal dominant pattern but is associated with an extra chromosome fragment. Colobomas may be associated with Wilms' tumour, but such cases are generally sporadic.

Heterochromia of the Iris
This is frequently an isolated and harmless trait, often autosomal dominant in inheritance. The most important cause of heterochromia to recognize is the Waardenburg syndrome, in which piebaldness and deafness are major features. Variation in expression of this autosomal dominant disorder is considerable.

Eye Colour
In Sheldon Reed's book, *Counselling in Medical Genetics* (1965), this is given as one of the most common reasons for requesting genetic counselling, but this seems rarely the case now. It is possible that such enquiries were really aimed at establishing paternity. In fact, while brown eye colour in general behaves as dominant to light blue eye colour, the genetic control is considerably more complex than this, and exceptions are sufficiently frequent for this trait *not* to be used as evidence for or against paternity.

Strabismus
This is a frequent feature of many generalized neuromuscular disorders, which may follow Mendelian inheritance. Isolated strabismus, whether classified as convergent or divergent, fits a polygenic pattern. Variation between studies results in part from the extent to which minor deviations are classed as abnormal. From the viewpoint of counselling it seems that where parents are normal and one child affected, the risk for subsequent children is around 15 per cent. Where one parent is also affected the risk is around 40 per cent.

Hereditary Ptosis
This is usually autosomal dominant and persists unchanged through life. Care must be taken to distinguish more general neuromuscular causes such as myotonic dystrophy.

Further Reading
Bergsma D., Bron A. J. and Cotlier E. (ed.) (1976) *The Eye and Inborn Errors of Metabolism.* New York, Alan Liss.

Goldberg M. F. (ed.) (1974) *Genetic and Metabolic Eye Disease.* Boston, Little, Brown.
Krill A. E. (1977) *Hereditary Retinal and Choroidal Diseases. Vol. 2. Clinical Characteristics.* Hagerstown, Harper & Row.
Sorsby A. (1970) *Ophthalmic Genetics.* London, Butterworth.
Waardenburg P. J., Franceschetti A. and Klein D. (1961) *Genetics and Ophthalmology.* Vols. 1 and 2. Assen, Royal Van Gorcum.

CHAPTER FIFTEEN

Deafness

A high proportion of deafness in children and young adults is genetically determined; reaching a precise genetic diagnosis may be exceedingly difficult and is often dependent on specialized audiologic testing. Close consultation with specialists in this field is needed if errors are to be avoided, and the author has found it helpful (and has learned much in the process) to hold a joint clinic for such families. Two groups particularly require genetic counselling: parents of a severely affected child wishing for further children, and young adults with deafness, who frequently marry partners similarly affected.

Table 15.1. Genetic risks in profound childhood deafness of unknown cause

Affected relative	Risk
One child only; environmental factors carefully excluded	1 in 6
One child only; consanguinity present	1 in 4
One affected child + 2 or more normal sibs	1 in 10
Two affected children	1 in 4
One parent + 1 child	1 in 2
One parent only	1 in 20
Parent + sib(s) of parent only	1 in 100
Sib(s) of parent; parent unaffected	<1 in 100

Even without access to specialized testing, it is often possible to assess the genetic situation accurately if the following points are borne in mind.

1. What does the pattern of inheritance in the particular family suggest?
2. Is the hearing loss severe congenital deafness, or some milder form?
3. If milder is it static or progressive?
4. Is there an identifiable syndrome involving other systems?

Further information on syndromes involving deafness and the classification of the various genetic forms of deafness can be found in the valuable book of Konigsmark and Gorlin, while a detailed study of profound childhood deafness is provided by Fraser.

Severe Congenital Sensorineural Deafness (deaf-mutism)

The incidence has been estimated to be around 1 in 1000 births. Care must be taken to exclude external factors such as mild congenital rubella or cytomegalovirus infection.

Where no clear environmental cause exists, there is no doubt that a high proportion of cases results from autosomal recessive inheritance. Exactly what proportion is difficult to decide since the different types are at present clinically indistinguishable. Most studies have suggested that 40–50 per cent of the cases are autosomal recessive, with around 10 per cent due to autosomal dominant inheritance and most of the rest due to unknown or undetected environmental (or at least non-Mendelian) factors. This would suggest that the risk of deafness in sibs of an isolated case is about 1 in 10; in fact it may well be higher than this, since studies suggesting this figure, such as that of Fraser (1976) were retrospective, and it is likely that intensive study might have distinguished more of the non-genetic cases. A risk of 1 in 6 for sibs of a thoroughly studied isolated case is probably appropriate. Where consanguinity exists, autosomal recessive inheritance is even more likely, and a 1 in 4 risk should be given. Likewise, should a couple have a second affected child, autosomal recessive inheritance is almost certain.

The risk for offspring of healthy sibs and other family members is often asked. This is extremely low (well under 1 per cent) in the absence of consanguinity or of deafness in the family of the other partner.

The risk for offspring of an affected individual who is an isolated case and married to a normal person is low, but not negligible (around 5 per cent). This risk probably results from an inclusion of unrecognized new dominant mutations with the much larger number following recessive inheritance. Where a parent and child are already affected, it is wise to assume autosomal dominant inheritance unless there is consanguinity, or other factors suggesting that a recessive gene may have been transmitted by the healthy parent. Although dominantly inherited severe congenital deafness is rare in comparison with recessive forms, it nevertheless accounts for the majority of two generation families. In families with two affected sibs and healthy parents, where recessive inheritance is almost certain, the risk for offspring of the affected individuals is low (around 1 per cent).

X-linked recessive inheritance is rare, but well-documented as a mode of inheritance in severe congenital deafness. It is not frequent enough to affect the risks for isolated male cases or single sibships containing only affected males.

Marriage between two individuals with severe congenital deafness is common, and the offspring of such matings provides clear evidence for the existence of several non-allelic recessive genes, probably 5–6 in number. If all cases were due to the same gene, or to different alleles at the same locus, one would expect all children to be affected. In fact, deaf children only occur in around 20 per cent of marriages between affected individuals and the risk of a pregnancy ending in a deaf child is only around 10 per cent; in around 70 per cent all children are unaffected, being heterozygous at each of the two loci involved. In only 5–10 per cent of marriages are all children affected; in the remainder, some children but not all prove to be affected, probably representing the situation where one of the partners has a dominant form of deafness. *Fig.* 15.1 shows the various possibilities, while *Table* 15.2 summarizes the risks for individual couples.

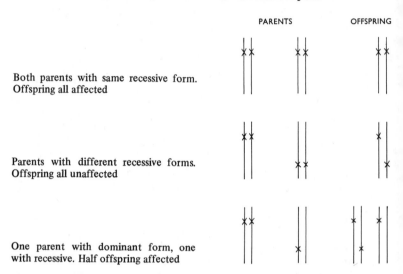

Fig. 15.1. Possibilities for marriages between congenitally deaf individuals.

Table 15.2. Risks for children of two parents with profound childhood deafness (risk for *next* child)

Number of children already born:	0	1 unaff.	1 aff.	2 aff.
Parents related	>1/2	1 in 10	1	1
Parents unrelated but from same minority ethnic group	> 1/2	1 in 10	1	1
Parents unrelated; not from same minority ethnic group	1 in 10	1 in 20	> 1/2	1

It is important to recognize that the risk for subsequent children of a couple may well be markedly altered by whether their first child proves to be affected or not, and this should be stressed when genetic counselling is given initially. Most couples are able to understand that the initial risk estimate is a provisional one, being made up of a high-risk and a low-risk element which cannot be distinguished until they have actually had a child. A deaf couple whose first child is also deaf have at least a 50 per cent chance of this occurring in the next pregnancy.

Partial Nerve Deafness

Into this large group fall numerous genetic forms of deafness whose effect is confined to the ear, but where hearing loss is not sufficient to present as 'congenital deaf mutism'. Some forms are present from birth and static, others later in onset and progressive, while detailed audiologic testing may show loss of particular frequencies. *Table* 15.3 lists some of the major types that can be recognized; it is likely that others will be delineated in future.

Table 15.3. Genetic forms of partial or progressive nerve deafness

	Onset	Progression	Severity	Other features
Autosomal dominant				
Dominant progressive nerve deafness	Childhood	Slow	Variable	High frequencies lost first
Dominant unilateral deafness	Birth	No	Severe	Occasionally bilateral
Dominant low-frequency deafness	Childhood	Slow	Variable	Low frequencies lost first
Dominant mild-frequency hearing loss	Childhood	Slow	Variable	Middle frequencies lost first
Autosomal recessive				
Recessive early onset nerve deafness	Infancy	Rapid	Severe	
Recessive congenital moderate deafness	Birth	No	Moderate	
X-linked recessive				
X-linked early onset deafness	Birth	Rapid	Moderate to severe	
X-linked moderate deafness	Childhood	Slow	Mild to moderate	High frequencies mainly lost

Several factors are especially relevant to genetic counselling in this group:

1. A considerably higher proportion of cases results from autosomal dominant inheritance than with severe congenital deafness.

2. Variability within a family can be considerable – careful testing is required before an individual is pronounced normal.

3. Isolated cases are extremely difficult to distinguish from non-genetic forms of hearing loss.

It can be seen that this is an extremely complex area; further information on the various subtypes is clearly set out in the monograph of Konigsmark and Gorlin.

Otosclerosis is the commonest disorder in this group and can be recognized by its progressive course and mixed conductive and neural pattern. It follows autosomal dominant inheritance with rather incomplete penetrance (around 40 per cent).

Deafness as part of Syndromes

Table 15.4 shows some of the large number that must be considered; they are particularly likely to be overlooked when the deafness is severe and the patient less likely to communicate complaints involving other systems.

Table 15.4. Syndromal associations with hereditary nerve deafness (based on Konigsmark and Gorlin)

Type	Inheritance	Type of hearing loss		
		Onset	Progression	Severity
Syndromes with skin disease				
Waardenburg's syndrome	Autosomal dominant	Birth	No	Variable
Hereditary piebaldness with deafness	Autosomal recessive	Birth	No	Moderate to severe
Cutaneous albinism with deafness	Autosomal dominant	Birth	No	Severe
Leopard syndrome	Autosomal dominant	Birth	No	Moderate to severe
Anhidrosis with progressive deafness	Autosomal dominant	Adult	Yes	Mild to moderate
Hyperkeratosis, digital constrictions and deafness	Autosomal dominant	Birth	No	Severe
Pili torti with deafness	Autosomal recessive	Birth	No	Moderate to severe
Knuckle pads, leukonychia and deafness	Autosomal dominant	Birth	Yes	Moderate to severe
Nail dystrophy with deafness	Autosomal recessive	Birth	No	Severe
Nail dystrophy, dental defects and deafness	Autosomal dominant	Birth	No	Moderate to severe
X-linked pigmentary defects and deafness	X recessive	Birth	No	Severe
Syndromes with eye disease				
Usher's syndrome (retinitis pigmentosa with deafness)	Autosomal recessive	Birth	No	Moderate to severe
Hallgren's syndrome (retinitis pigmentosa, vestibular ataxia and deafness)	Autusomal recessive	Birth	No	Severe
Myopia with congenital deafness	Autosomal recessive	Birth	No	Moderate to severe
Stickler's syndrome (*see* p. 168)	Autosomal dominant	Childhood	Yes	Moderate to severe
Refsum's syndrome	Autosomal recessive	Childhood or older	Yes	Variable
Alström's syndrome (diabetes, deafness and retinal degeneration)	Autosomal recessive	Childhood	Yes	Moderate
Optic atrophy, diabetes and deafness	Autosomal recessive	Childhood	Yes	Moderate

| Type | Inheritance | Type of hearing loss | | |
		Onset	Progression	Severity
Corneal dystrophy with deafness	Autosomal dominant	Adult	Yes	Moderate
Mental subnormality with ataxia, deafness and hypogonadism	Autosomal recessive	Infancy	Yes	Moderate to severe
Myoclonus with deafness, diabetes and nephropathy	Autosomal dominant	Adult	Yes	Moderate
Sensory radicular neuropathy	Autosomal dominant	Early adult	Yes	Moderate to severe
Bilateral acoustic neuromas	Autosomal dominant	Early adult	Yes	Moderate to severe
Syndromes with other systems				
Alport's disease (hereditary nephropathy with deafness)	?X-linked recessive	Late Childhood	Yes	Mild to moderate
Nephropathy with deafness and ichthyosis	Autosomal dominant	Childhood	Yes	Mild to moderate
Amyloidosis, deafness and nephropathy	Autosomal dominant	Late Childhood	Yes	Mild to moderate
Pendred's syndrome	Autosomal recessive	Birth	No	Moderate to severe
Deafness with cardiac defect	Autosomal recessive	Birth	No	Severe

Three syndromes (all autosomal recessive) are of especial importance since they are considerably commoner than the others and have serious consequences if overlooked. These are:

1. Pendred's syndrome: Severe nerve deafness with goitrous hypothyroidism; early thyroxine treatment is important here.

2. Jervell—Nielsen syndrome: Severe nerve deafness with abnormal cardiac conduction. Sudden death may occur.

3. Usher's syndrome: Severe nerve deafness with retinitis pigmentosa.

The External Ear

Several syndromes, both dominantly and recessively inherited, have been described in which deafness, usually conductive, has been associated with abnormal shape of the external ear as the only visible feature.

External ear malformation is also striking in the Goldenhar syndrome, mandibulofacial dysostosis and the Wildervanck syndrome of deafness, malformed ears and vertebral defects. This last disorder is seen mainly in females and it is uncertain whether it follows autosomal dominant inheritance or whether it is an X-linked dominant lethal in the male. Environmental causes include rubella and thalidomide embryopathies and the 'Potter facies' resulting from oligohydramnios secondary to renal agenesis. Lesser degrees of abnormality form part of the characteristic facies of many genetic syndromes.

Isolated external ear abnormalities, particularly when unilateral, carry a low recurrence risk, but a careful examination should be carried out for minor audiological or branchial arch defects on both sides.

Menière's Disease

A few familial aggregations of this common disorder have been recorded, but one can safely say that the risks to family members of a single case are low.

Further Reading

Fraser G. R. (1976) *The Causes of Profound Deafness in Childhood.* Baltimore, Johns Hopkins University Press.

Konigsmark B. W. and Gorlin R. J. (1976) *Genetic and Metabolic Deafness.* Philadelphia, Saunders.

CHAPTER SIXTEEN

Cardiovascular Diseases

Heart disease provides a large number of genetic counselling problems and, fortunately, has been well studied from the viewpoint of recurrence risks and underlying aetiology. Congenital heart disease is the largest group for which advice is asked, usually regarding the risks for further affected children, but increasingly concerning the offspring of a successfully treated patient. The monograph by Nora and Nora provides an excellent synthesis of our current knowledge on the subject, as well as a detailed source of literature on individual defects.

Paradoxically, coronary heart disease, the largest single cause of death in Western populations, is less frequently encountered as a counselling problem, in part because its commonness means it is a problem for everybody, in part because of a somewhat fatalistic acceptance of a high risk in those families where early coronary disease is concentrated. In view of our confused state of knowledge, it is perhaps fortunate that precise risk figures are not often requested.

Congenital Heart Disease
Congenital heart disease occurs in around 1 per cent of births; most, probably as much as 90 per cent, is of unknown aetiology and is classed as 'polygenic'; only around 3 per cent of cases follow Mendelian inheritance. None the less, the first task in genetic counselling of families is to ensure that a Mendelian disorder has been excluded, particularly if other abnormalities than the cardiac lesion are present. *Table* 16.1 lists some of the more important Mendelian syndromes characterized by cardiac involvement that must be distinguished. Congenital heart disease is also prominent in chromosomal disorders, particularly the autosomal trisomies and Turner's syndrome, while there are a number of looser associations which do not follow Mendelian inheritance (*Table* 16.2).

Among the identified environmental causes, rubella is the most important, but congenital heart defects are produced by almost all the less specific teratogens and environmental factors should be carefully enquired for, even though it may not be possible to prove cause and effect in an individual case. The offspring of diabetic women also appear to be a high risk group (*see* Chapter 17). Some increase of congenital heart disease with maternal age has been shown (excluding Down's syndrome). A risk of

Table 16.1. Heart disease in Mendelian disorders

Disorder	Main extracardiac features	Usual heart defects	Inheritance
Holt–Oram syndrome	Upper limb defects, especially digits and radius	Atrial septal defect	AD
Ellis–van Creveld syndrome	Dwarfism, mid-line cleft lip, polydactyly	Ventricular septal defect	AR
Noonan's syndrome	'Turner like' phenotype	Pulmonary stenosis	? variable AD
Marfan's syndrome	Skeletal abnormalities, lens dislocation	Septal defect; valve prolapse	AD
Supravalvular aortic stenosis syndrome	Mental retardation, unusual facies, hypercalcaemia	Supravalvular aortic stenosis	? variable AD
Obstructive cardio-myopathy	—		? variable AD
Leopard syndrome ?	Nerve deafness, lentigenes	Conduction defects	AD
Q–T (Romano–Ward) syndrome	—	Conduction defects (prolonged Q–T)	AD
Kartagener's syndrome	Situs inversus	Dextrocardia	? AR
Jervell–Nielsen syndrome	Nerve deafness	Congenital conduction defects	AR

AD, autosomal dominant; AR, autosomal recessive.

Table 16.2. Non-Mendelian syndromes with congenital heart disease

Disorder	Non-cardiac features	Cardiac lesion
Asplenia and polysplenia syndromes	Complex lateralized defects	Dextrocardia and other complex defects
'VATER' syndrome	Oesophageal, anal, vertebral and radial limb defects	Variable
Klippel–Feil syndrome	Fusion and reduction of cervical vertebrae	Cardiac involvement (commonly septal defects) in at least 1/4
Di George's syndrome	Absent thymus and parathyroids	VSD and other defects in 75%
Goldenhar's syndrome	Eye, ear and facial abnormalities	Various defects in half

around 2 per cent (twice that for the general population) is appropriate for women aged 40 or more.

Genetic advice is most frequently asked for future sibs of an affected child, or sometimes for more distant relatives; information is now becoming available for the offspring of affected individuals and so far shows risks comparable to those of sibs, supporting the view that polygenic inheritance is operating. Unlike some other polygenic disorders, there is no marked sex difference in incidence or in risk estimates. Overall risks are summarized in *Table* 16.3. Wherever possible a specific anatomical diagnosis should be used as the basis for risk estimates, and data for a

Table 16.3. Overall risks in congenital heart disease

	Risk (%)
Population incidence	1
Sibs of isolated case	2
Offspring of isolated case	3
Two affected sibs (or sib + parent)	10
More than two affected first-degree relatives	50

Table 16.4. Genetic risks in congenital heart disease

Disorder	Incidence (per 1000 live births)	Recurrence risk % (after isolated case)	
		Sibs	Offspring
VSD	2·5−5	2·1−4·2 (3)	4·0
ASD	1·0	2·9−3·7 (3)	2·5
Patent ductus	0·5−1·2	1·0−3·5 (3)	1·7−4·3 (3)
Fallot's tetralogy	0·7	3·0	4·2
A−V canal defect	0·7	2·6	
Pulmonary stenosis	0·8	1·5−2·7 (2)	3·6
Aortic stenosis	0·5	2·2	3·9
Coarctation	0·15	1·0−1·8	2·7
Transposition of great vessels	0·4	1·7	
Pulmonary atresia	0·2	1·3	
Common truncus	0·15	1·2	
Tricuspid atresia	0·15	1·0	
Ebstein's anomaly	0·12	1·0	
Hypoplastic left heart	0·2	2·7	
Endocardial fibroelastosis	0·17	3·8	

Risk estimates are for all forms of congenital heart disease. Data mainly from Nora and Spangler[14] and Nora and Nora (1978)
Figures in brackets represent a reasonable figure to use in counselling where series vary considerably.

number of the more common defects are given in *Table* 16.4. Where recurrence does occur, the defect is the same as previously in only about one-half the cases; this is relevant to counselling since it may mean that a sib of a proband with a correctable defect may have a fatal or untreatable lesion, or vice versa.

A number of particular problems are encountered:

1. The affected individual is dead, with no precise diagnosis as to the type of defect. Here, one is forced to use the overall risk of 2 per cent, but

families should understand that the true risk will be between 1 and 4 per cent.

2. The defect is rare and there are no satisfactory data. Fortunately, the recurrence risk approximates to the square root of the incidence (*see* Chapter 3), and is unlikely to exceed 1 per cent for really rare defects.

3. A combination of cardiac defects exists. Apart from specific combinations, such as Fallot's tetralogy, it is probably wise to use the risk for the most frequent individual component.

Risks to More Distant Relatives

Data are inadequate but the risk for second-degree relatives of an isolated case is certainly under 1 per cent and it is doubtful if third-degree relatives have a significantly raised risk. Families are not infrequently encountered where there are several affected members, none of whom are first-degree relatives; computerized risk prediction has been attempted to help in this situation, but in practice one usually sums the various individual risks.

Multiple Cases

Family clusters of congenital heart disease are not uncommon; their occurrence should prompt a careful search for a Mendelian syndrome or teratogenic factor, but in most cases this proves negative. After two affected children the risk of congenital heart disease in future sibs is approximately trebled, regardless of whether the affected individuals have the same heart defect or not. This gives risks ranging from 5 per cent for the rarer defects to 10 per cent for a common abnormality such as VSD. A similar risk would be likely for future children where an affected parent has an affected child, though data to confirm this are not yet available. Numbers are insufficient to give individual estimates for specific defects. The occurrence of more distant affected relatives does not greatly raise the risks given in *Table* 16.4. In the occasional families with more than two affected first-degree relatives, risks are likely to be extremely high, even though the factors underlying such occurrences are not understood.

Atrial Septal Defect (ASD)

The recurrence risk is around 3 per cent for sibs and 2·5 per cent for offspring of an isolated case. Occasional families following autosomal dominant inheritance probably exist, as well as dominant syndromal associations such as the Holt–Oram syndrome and ASD with AV conduction defects. These families are too rare to affect the general recurrence risks, but should be borne in mind when familial clusters of three or more patients are encountered, which should probably be counselled as Mendelian.

Ventricular Septal Defect

A 3 per cent recurrence risk for sibs is appropriate, allowing for the variation between different series. The figures given apply to severe defects, mostly those patients requiring surgery. It is doubtful whether the risks are as high for relatives of patients with asymptomatic or transient defects. The recurrence risk after two affected children is around 10 per cent, and for offspring of an affected parent, 4 per cent.

Patent Ductus Arteriosus
Congenital rubella must be excluded. The recurrence risk varies considerably between series (*Table* 16.4) but 3 per cent seems a reasonable figure for both sibs and offspring.

Endocardial Fibroelastosis
This may be secondary to acquired myocarditis or may accompany other congenital heart defects. Idiopathic fibroelastosis should only be accepted as the diagnosis with autopsy evidence. A thorough study from Toronto[1] has shown a recurrence risk of 3·8 per cent in sibs, rather higher than expected from the incidence of the disorder. It is possible that a small subgroup follows autosomal recessive inheritance, but if it exists it cannot be distinguished from the majority at present.

Hypoplastic Left Heart Syndrome
Shokeir has suggested autosomal recessive inheritance[2], but his families may well have been ascertained because of multiple affected members. A more systematic study[3] has shown a low risk of congenital heart disease in sibs (2·7 per cent), comparable to other congenital heart defects.

Dextrocardia with Asplenia
Absence of the spleen – or the presence of multiple spleens – is an important point to note at autopsy in congenital heart disease, since a combination of defects involving left-sided visceral structures is seen with asplenia, and a corresponding series involving right-sided ones with polysplenia. The recurrence risk seems negligible so it is important to distinguish these cases, with various cardiac defects, especially dextrocardia, from other types of congenital heart disease. The only high risk association with dextrocardia is Kartagener's syndrome (*see* p. 211).

Noonan's Syndrome (Turner phenotype with normal chromosomes)
The characteristic facies with ptosis and low set ears, as well as the different cardiac defect (pulmonary stenosis) from that of Turner's syndrome, should allow clinical recognition of this relatively common disorder in either sex. Autosomal dominant inheritance has been suggested on the basis of cases of parent-child transmission (*see* Nora and Nora, 1978, for discussion). However, the features in the parent have usually been mild and rather unconvincing. The risk to sibs of an isolated case is low.

Williams' Syndrome (Hypercalcaemia with supravalvular aortic stenosis and unusual facies)
Many cases are isolated and some have been related to excessive maternal vitamin D intake. A number of families appear to follow autosomal dominant inheritance, though not all members have complete expression of the syndrome. Counselling as for autosomal dominance is wise in any case with affected relatives; the risk for sibs of an isolated case is probably 10 per cent at most. It seems sensible for mothers at risk to avoid vitamin D in pregnancy.

Cardiomyopathies
These may form part of primary Mendelian disorders such as Type II glycogenosis, Duchenne and myotonic dystrophy, and Friedreich's ataxia.

Obstructive cardiomyopathy appears to be inherited as a variable autosomal dominant; penetrance is near complete if the family is studied by echocardiography, but only around 25 per cent clinically, i.e. there is a risk of 1 in 8 for clinical disease in first-degree relatives.

Other less well-defined cardiomyopathies may be familial and until they are better understood, genetic advice is best based on the observed family pattern.

Congenital Conduction Defects
Most cases are isolated, but familial forms to be considered include the Jervell–Nielsen syndrome (AR) with deafness, the dominantly inherited prolonged Q–T syndrome with sudden death, and the occurrence of complete heart-block in offspring of mothers with systemic lupus erythematosus. In isolated congenital complete heart block a recurrence risk of 2–5 per cent has been found in sibs.

Coronary Heart Disease
The epidemic increase of coronary heart disease in recent decades, now possibly declining, is likely to be environmentally caused, but it is probable that susceptibility has a strong genetic basis, particularly when onset is early. Two particular influences have been identified.
   a. The major gene of familial hypercholesterolaemia and other genetic influences on lipid levels.
   b. Polygenic factors independent of lipid status.

Familial hypercholesterolaemia (Type II hyperlipoproteinaemia) should be suspected whenever a familial aggregation of early coronary heart disease occurs. Many patients will show xanthomas or other cholesterol deposits, but vascular disease may be the only clinical feature. It is most important to recognize that the great majority of lipid abnormalities found in such patients are secondary to dietary factors or other disorders and that Type II hyperlipoproteinaemia should only be diagnosed when these have been excluded. Even when only primary cases with typical lipoprotein abnormalities are considered, it seems likely that the majority are multifactorial in their origin, rather than following Mendelian inheritance. Classic familial hypercholesterolaemia, accounting for around 10 per cent of early coronary heart disease, is an autosomal dominant disorder, with a heterozygote prevalence estimated to be around 1 in 400 to 1 in 1000. Affected homozygotes with severe childhood disease are well recognized but extremely rare. The risk of offspring of a heterozygous patient inheriting the gene is of course 50 per cent, but the risk of heart disease, which is the relevant factor, is considerably less than this, particularly in females[4] (*Table* 16.5). The risk to offspring of an isolated case showing this lipid abnormality is also considerably less than where an established dominant pattern exists in the family, since a proportion of the non-genetic lipid defects are indistinguishable from it.

The gene can be reliably detected in early childhood by lipoprotein electrophoresis, and possibly in cord blood by analysis of low-density lipoprotein cholesterol. The basic defect has been established in fibroblasts as a receptor deficiency[5], or in some families an alteration of the receptor, and the homozygous form (but not the heterozygote) can be diagnosed prenatally[6].

Table 16.5. Risks of heart disease in familial hypercholesterolaemia (after Slack)[4]

Age (years)	Per cent with ischaemic heart disease Males	Females
30	5·4	0
30–39	23·7	0
40–49	51·4	12·2
50–59	85·4	57·5
60–69	100	74·4

Table 16.6. Risk of death from ischaemic heart disease between age 35–55 in first degree relatives of index patients with ischaemic heart disease. (From Slack and Evans[7]. Increase over general population incidence given in brackets

	Male index case	Female index case
Male first-degree relative	1 in 12 (X 5)	1 in 10 (X 6½)
Female first-degree relative	1 in 36 (X 2½)	1 in 12 (X 7)

Other Genetic Influences on Coronary Heart Disease

The risk of death from ischaemic heart disease in relatives of patients with ischaemic heart disease has been studied by Slack and Evans[7], who found a marked increase for all groups of first-degree relatives (*Table* 16.6). As expected the increase is greater where the index patient was female (*see*

Chapter 3) though the absolute risk figure is greater for male relatives than for females. A few families with hypercholesterolaemia were included in this study, but do not significantly affect the risks.

Familial aggregations of early coronary heart disease are encountered in which there is no detectable lipid abnormality nor any other primary cause that can be identified. Some of these are strikingly suggestive of autosomal dominant inheritance, and where a pattern of this type is seen it is wise to give risks accordingly for the offspring of affected individuals, and to ensure that their risk is reduced as far as is possible by appropriate preventive measures. It is likely that specific genetic loci will be identified in the near future. Some rare causes of premature vascular disease are listed in *Table* 16.7 but account for only a small proportion of the total problem.

Table 16.7. Some rare genetic causes of premature vascular disease

Disorder	Inheritance
Pseudoxanthoma elasticum	Autosomal recessive (sometimes AD)
Homocystinuria	Autosomal recessive
Progeria	Autosomal recessive
Cockayne's syndrome	Autosomal recessive
Werner's syndrome	Autosomal recessive
Menkes' syndrome	X-linked recessive

Hypertension

There is general agreement that there is an important genetic contribution to essential hypertension; earlier debate as to whether this was polygenic or involved major genes has subsided since it became clear that the two positions were not incompatible. However, no identifiable specific genes have yet been recognized, nor are there precise figures on which to base genetic advice. It is sensible for first-degree relatives, particularly in a family with multiple affected members, to be aware of their increased risk so that early treatment can be started if required and aggravating factors avoided.

Lymphatic Disorders

Mild lymphoedema of hands and feet may be seen in both Turner's and Noonan's syndromes. The commonest and most severe form of lymphoedema, *Milroy's syndrome*, follows autosomal dominant inheritance, and can usually be recognized at birth. A milder and later onset form (Meige's syndrome) is more variable in inheritance. It is uncertain at present whether the pattern is autosomal recessive or autosomal dominant with variable penetrance.

Two specific autosomal dominant syndromes are lymphoedema with yellow nails, and lymphoedema with distichiasis (double eyelashes).

Rheumatic Fever

The recognition of a streptococcal basis for this disorder and its dramatic decline in Western populations should not obscure the fact that susceptibility is strongly influenced by inheritance. Early studies[8] showed a risk of around 10 per cent in sibs and offspring of an affected person developing the condition at some later stage of life, and double this when a parent and a sib were affected. The risks are now likely to represent susceptibility rather than actual disease, but may still be appropriate for the many parts of the world where the disorder remains common.

Pulmonary Disease

Surprisingly few pulmonary disorders show a clear pattern of inheritance. Two important autosomal recessive disorders, *cystic fibrosis* and α_1-*antitrypsin deficiency*, are discussed in Chapter 17. There is no evidence that the heterozygotes in either condition are more prone to common lung diseases.

Microcystic disease of the lung is a rare disorder which also follows autosomal recessive inheritance.

Kartagener's syndrome, characterized by bronchiectasis, recurrent sinusitis, dextrocardia and other heart defects, and often asplenia, has traditionally been considered autosomal recessive. Recent work has shown this disorder to be part of a more extensive group of defects of cilial function[9], often accompanied by male infertility. A family study has shown a recurrence risk in sibs of 13 per cent, but no transmission to children[10], which would fit well with autosomal recessive inheritance and penetrance of 1/2.

Sarcoidosis is occasionally familial, but affected members are usually related in the maternal line[11]. Satisfactory risk figures do not appear to exist.

Bronchial asthma is commonly familial when 'extrinsic' in type and associated with atopy and a recent study has shown 13 per cent of first-degree relatives affected in this group, while the risk was only 5 per cent for first-degree relatives of intrinsic cases[12].

Lung cancer has long been recognized to have a genetic predisposition, interacting with environmental factors, and the discovery of association with aryl carbon hydroxylase levels probably provides the basis of this[13]. Genetic counselling is of little relevance in the face of obvious environmental causes.

Familial stridor, resulting from congenital laryngeal muscle palsies of several types commonly follows autosomal dominant inheritance.

References

1. Chen S., Thompson M. W. and Rose V. (1971) Endocardial fibroelastosis. Family studies with special reference to counseling. *J. Pediatr.* 79, 385–392.
2. Shokeir M. H. K. (1971) Hypoplastic left heart syndrome. An autosomal recessive disorder. *Clin. Genet.* 2, 7–14.
3. Holmes L. B., Rose V., Child A. H. et al. (1974) Hypoplastic left heart. Comments. In: Bergsma D. (ed.), *Clinical Delineation of Birth Defects. Part 15*. Baltimore, Williams & Wilkins, pp. 228–229.
4. Slack J. (1969) Risks of ischaemic heart disease in familial hyperlipoproteinaemic states. *Lancet* 2, 1380–1382.
5. Brown M. S. and Goldstein J. L. (1974) Familial hypercholesterolaemia. Defective binding of lipoproteins to cultured fibroblasts associated with impaired regulation of HMG COA reductase activity. *Proc. Natl Acad. Sci. USA* 71, 788–792.
6. Brown M. S., Goldstein J. L., Vandenberghe K. et al. (1978) Prenatal diagnosis of homozygous familial hypercholesterolaemia. *Lancet* 1, 526–529.
7. Slack J. and Evans K. A. (1966) The increased risk of death from ischaemic heart disease in first degree relatives of 121 men and 96 women with ischaemic heart disease. *J. Med. Genet.* 3, 239–257.
8. Wilson M. G. and Schweitzer M. D. (1954) Pattern of hereditary susceptibility in rheumatic fever. Circulation 10, 699–704.
9. Afzelius B. A. (1976) A human syndrome caused by immotile cilia. *Science* 193, 317–319.
10. Child A. H. (1980) Kartagener's syndrome, a family study. *Clin. Genet.* 17, 61.
11. Sharma O. P., Neville E., Walker A. N. et al. (1976) Familial sarcoidosis: a possible genetic influence. *Ann. NY Acad. Sci.* 278, 386–400.
12. Sibbald B. and Turner-Warwick M. (1979) Factors influencing the prevalence of asthma among first degree relatives of extrinsic and intrinsic asthmatics. *Thorax* 34, 332–337.
13. Emery A. E. H., Anad R., Danford N. et al. (1978) Aryl-hydrocarbon hydroxylase inducibility in patients with cancer. *Lancet* 1, 470–471.
14. Nora J. J. and Spangler R. D. (1972) Risks and counseling in cardiovascular malformations. In: Bergsma D. (ed.), *Clinical Delineation of Birth Defects. Part 15*. Baltimore, Williams & Wilkins, pp. 154–159.

Further Reading

Bergsma D. (1972) *Clinical Delineation of Birth Defects. Part 15, The cardiovascular system*. Baltimore, Williams & Wilkins.

McKusick V. A. (1972) *Heritable Disorders of Connective Tissue*. St. Louis, Mosby.

Nora J. J. and Nora A. H. (1978) *Genetics and Counseling in Cardiovascular Diseases*. Springfield, Thomas.

CHAPTER SEVENTEEN

The Gastrointestinal Tract

Relatively few gastrointestinal disorders follow Mendelian inheritance, so that genetic counselling is more dependent on empiric risks than is the case for some other systems. Most data of this type have been collected for Western European or American populations, so figures must be applied with caution in other areas, particularly where the incidence of the disorder is known to differ significantly from the usual level.

Gastrointestinal disorders have also proved more treatable than most groups, so that individuals with previously fatal disorders now reproduce. Data for such risks are available for only a few conditions such as pyloric stenosis, and in preliminary form for Hirschsprung's disease and oesophageal atresia.

Oesophageal Atresia

Most cases are combined with tracheo-oesophageal fistula. As many as 55 per cent of cases have been found to be associated with other malformations, notably rectal and duodenal atresia, diaphragmatic hernia, hypoplasia of the radius and renal agenesis. Despite this, the recurrence risk to sibs in a large series of 345 patients[1] was very low (1 affected sib), so the presence of associated defects (unless part of a specific syndrome) should not be grounds for giving a higher risk. Risk figures for offspring of treated patients are becoming available, and appear to be low, probably not more than 1 per cent[34].

Oesophageal Cancer

The risk to relatives is not obviously increased, at least in Western Europe [2]. The situation may be different in high incidence areas such as Central Asia and parts of Africa, where striking family clusters have been reported [3]. Environmental factors are probably responsible for the major differences in incidence. The remarkable, but exceedingly rare families with oesophageal cancer and tylosis (hyperkeratosis of palms and soles) following autosomal dominant inheritance[4, 5] should be borne in mind if a family cluster is found in a low incidence area.

Diaphragmatic Hernia

Although a few instances of affected sibs, most with complete aplasia of the diaphragm, have been reported[6], the overall risk is extremely low, certainly less than 1 per cent. David and Illingworth[7] found no affected sibs in a series from South-West England, though half the cases had associated defects, most commonly of the nervous system. Diaphragmatic hypoplasia is seen in some primary myopathies (e.g. congenital myotonic dystrophy).

Hiatus hernia, whether in infancy or adult life does not seem to show any notable increase in incidence in relatives.

Infantile Pyloric Stenosis

This disorder follows the pattern expected for polygenic inheritance, with risks diminishing rapidly outside first-degree relatives, and with relatives of index patients of the more rarely affected sex (female) having a higher risk. There is evidence for the action of an intrauterine environmental factor and possibly for an X-linked modifying gene. The most extensive study of risks is that from England of Carter and Evans[8], whose data are summarized in *Table* 17.1. Data are also available from Northern Ireland,

Table 17.1. Risks to relatives of patients with infantile pyloric stenosis (after Carter and Evans, 1969).

| | *Male index patients* | | *Female index patients* | |
	Risk (%)	Increase	Risk (%)	Increase
Brothers	3·8	X 8	9·2	X 18
Sisters	2·7	X 27	3·8	X 38
Sons	5·5	X 11	18·9	X 38
Daughters	2·4	X 24	7·0	X 70
Nephews	2·3	X4·6	4·7	X9·4
Nieces	0·4	X3·6	–	–
Male first cousins	0·9	X1·9	0·7	X1·3
Female first cousins	0·2	X2·3	0·3	X2·6

where Dodge[9] found a higher risk to male sibs of male index patients (9·4 per cent), but similar risks otherwise to those of Carter and Evans.

The overall population incidence for Britain is around 3 per 1000 births (5 per 1000 male births and 1 per 1000 female births). Data on risks for families with more than one affected individual are not available.

Omphalocele and Exomphalos

The Beckwith syndrome of exomphalos, macroglossia, general somatic overgrowth and hypoglycaemia is an important and treatable cause to exclude. The few familial cases of this syndrome have been either sibs or have been related in the maternal line[10].

Isolated omphalocele has a low (under 1 per cent) recurrence risk in sibs[11] though a few clusters have been reported[12]. Severe cases may be detected prenatally by a raised amniotic fluid or serum alphafetoprotein;

this is most commonly an incidental occurence in a pregnancy tested for other reasons.

Bowel Atresias and Malrotations
Most cases are sporadic. Meconium ileus from cystic fibrosis must be excluded as a cause of atresia. A recessively inherited form of malrotation associated with short mesentery (so called 'apple peel' syndrome) has also been recorded[13]. Duodenal atresia occurs with increased frequency in Down's syndrome.

Peptic Ulcer
Genetic studies are difficult in a disorder which is both common (around 4 per cent of adult males and 2 per cent of adult females in Britain) and where symptoms are often ill-defined. McConnell[14] gives a full discussion of the early work and known genetic factors. Most surveys have shown

Table 17.2. Risks to relatives of patients with duodenal ulcer (proven cases only) (from Cowan[15])

Relative	Risk (%)	Control prevalence (%)
First degree	10·5	1·7
Second degree	7·4	2·0
Third degree	3·5	1·2

around a threefold increase in both sibs and offspring. Childhood cases more commonly have an affected relative. Gastric and duodenal ulcer tend to run separately in families and people of blood group O are 35 per cent more liable than others to duodenal ulcer. Cowan[15] gives valuable data on the risks to relatives of patients with duodenal ulcer in Northern England; his figures for *proven* cases are given in *Table* 17.2, and include control series. When divided by sex the risk for male relatives was 2·5 × that for females.

Gastric Cancer
As with oesophageal cancer there are considerable geographical variations in incidence, in which genetic factors may play a part (e.g. in the Welsh) [16]. No clear Mendelian form has been described, though there are some notable family aggregations, the most famous being that of Napoleon Bonaparte. A modest 2—4 fold increase has been shown in first-degree relatives of patients[17].

Atrophic Gastritis and Pernicious Anaemia
One-quarter of first-degree relatives of patients with atrophic gastritis have histological evidence of the disorder; a similar proportion shows parietal cell antibodies[18]. A family study of patients with pernicious anaemia

[19] has shown parietal cell antibodies in half the sibs, with a quarter showing achlorhydria. It seems likely that an autosomal dominant gene controlling production of autoantibodies is involved; there is extensive overlap with other autoimmune disorders and autoantibodies within families.

Coeliac Disease

The risks to relatives depend on the thoroughness with which they are investigated and the criteria for diagnosis. Early studies showed an incidence of overt disease in sibs of 6—12 per cent, while later series using jejunal biopsy [20, 21] showed close agreement at around 10 per cent for both sibs and offspring. One study has given a much higher risk (18 per cent)[22], but in view of the close agreement of the other series 10 per cent would seem the soundest estimate for first-degree relatives. Risks to second-degree or more distant relatives appear small, not exceeding 1 per cent for overt disease.

Utilization of the association between coeliac disease and HLA B8 antigen does not appear to be helpful in risk prediction[23] but the much stronger association with DW3 has yet to be evaluated from this angle.

Gastrointestinal Enzyme Defects

These all follow autosomal recessive inheritance and include

1. Disaccharidase deficiencies (maltase, sucrase, lactase). Partial lactase deficiency after infancy is normal in many Eastern and African populations.

2. Pancreatic enzyme deficiencies (trypsinogen, enterokinase, lipase).

3. Acrodermatitis enteropathica (possibly due to a defect in zinc metabolism).

Intussusception

A risk of 1 in 40 to sibs of childhood cases has been shown as compared with 1 in 750 for the general population[24].

Inflammatory Bowel Disease

Overlap within families has been shown between ulcerative colitis and Crohn's disease[25]. Recurrence risks are low in both disorders, being estimated at between 1 in 250 and 1 in 100 for first-degree relatives of patients with Crohn's disease (prevalence around 1 in 5000). No accurate risks exist for ulcerative colitis (prevalence around 1 in 1500) but they are unlikely to exceed 1 per cent for first-degree relatives. A lethal form of enterocolitis in infancy has been described which apparently follows autosomal recessive inheritance[26]. It may well prove to have a metabolic basis.

Intestinal Polyposis

At least four separate genetic disorders exist in this group[17]:

1. Polyposis coli — autosomal dominant inheritance, with penetrance 80—90 per cent[27], and very high incidence of malignancy if colectomy

is not performed. Regular supervision of first-degree relatives is essential to prevent cancer developing, and the disorder is suitable for central registration. The incidence is around 1 in 7500.

2. The Gardner syndrome (autosomal dominant). Here a variety of soft-tissue and bone tumours (usually benign) accompany the polyposis. The risk of colonic cancer is high and the management is similar to polyposis coli.

3. Peutz—Jeghers syndrome (autosomal dominant). Characterized externally by circumoral pigment spots, polyps and neoplasms may occur throughout the gastrointestinal tract. The risk of malignancy is less than in polyposis coli but is considerable and less preventable owing to the wider distribution of lesions.

4. Discrete solitary colonic polyps. A few families following autosomal dominant inheritance have been reported.

Colonic Cancer
A very few families have been described following a pattern strongly suggesting autosomal dominant inheritance, but with no evidence of polyposis. A few others are part of the 'adenocarcinomatosis syndrome' (*see* Chapter 22). Apart from these the risks to relatives of a patient with colonic cancer are low (two to five-fold increase for first-degree relatives). The risk may be higher where tumours are multiple or early in onset[17].

Table 17.3. Genetic risks to sibs in Hirschsprung's disease (based on Passarge[28])

		Brothers (%)	Sisters (%)
All lengths of aganglionic segment	Male index patient	5·3	2·3
	Female index patient	11·3	13·6
Short aganglionic segment	Male index patient	4·7	0·6
	Female index patient	8·1	2·9
Long aganglionic segment	Male index patient	16·1	11·1
	Female index patient	18·2	9·1

Hirschsprung's Disease
The risks depend on the sex of index patient and relative, and on the length of the aganglionic segment, as is to be expected in polygenic inheritance. The male : female ratio of patients is around 3 : 1, and long segment involvement makes up 13 per cent of all cases. The overall population incidence is about 1 in 5000 births (0·02 per cent).

Table 17.3 is taken (with some revision) from the review of Passarge [28], and combines the three major family studies. Risks for offspring of affected patients with short segment disease, are now becoming available (Carter and Evans, personal communication) and are low, probably not over 1 per cent. Risks for second- and third-degree relatives are imprecise but are low.

Imperforate Anus
This is seen in various syndromes, notably with ocular coloboma in association with an extra chromosome fragment[29] (*see* Chapter 4), and with vertebral and radial limb defects (*see* Chapter 11). There is no evidence of a high recurrence risk to sibs either in the VATER syndrome or in isolated imperforate anus.

Hereditary Pancreatitis
Inheritance is autosomal dominant with penetrance around 80 per cent. This is a rare but important cause of recurrent abdominal pain in childhood[30]. Type V hyperlipoproteinaemia (autosomal recessive) may also cause recurrent pancreatitis.

Cystic Fibrosis
Although this is the commonest autosomal recessive disorder in Western Europe and in White Americans, the basic defect remains so far (1980) unknown. The incidence is around 1 in 2000 births, with a carrier frequency of 1 in 22; risks to offspring of patients and healthy sibs can be calculated as in *Table* 2.2 (p. 33). The incidence in Jewish, Asiatic and African populations is considerably lower. No reliable methods of carrier detection or prenatal diagnosis are yet available, despite numerous (and conflicting) reports on the subject. Nor is it known whether genetic heterogeneity exists. At a clinical level a wide range of severity may occur in a single sibship. Newborn screening (using meconium albumin content) detects only a minority of cases; blood trypsin on a filter paper blood spot is being assessed at present. Heterozygotes are entirely healthy. The Schwachman syndrome, in which pancreatic insufficiency is accompanied by bone marrow hypoplasia and, less constantly, a metaphyseal bone dysplasia, is also autosomal recessive in inheritance.

Metabolic Liver Disease
Liver involvement occurs in numerous metabolic disorders, including lipidoses, mucopolysaccharidoses, glycogenoses and galactosaemia. A few require separate mention.
  1. Wilson's disease (autosomal recessive). Prenatal diagnosis and carrier detection are not possible.
  2. Haemochromatosis. Autosomal recessive, but largely sex-limited to males[31]; heterozygotes show mild and usually clinically insignificant iron storage in most families. Transmission of the full disease by an affected person is very rare, but sibs have a 1 in 4 risk (clinical onset delayed and reduced in females). A close HLA linkage has been found which should help prediction of which sibs will be affected[32].
  3. α_1-antitrypsin deficiency. Incidence 1 in 2000 to 1 in 4000 (autosomal recessive). This is an important cause of neonatal hepatitis and cirrhosis. Some adults develop emphysema; others remain healthy. Heterozygotes are detectable and healthy. Prenatal diagnosis is not feasible at

present. Numerous harmless polymorphic variants of the protein also exist and must not be confused with the actual deficiency.

Hyperbilirubinaemias
This heterogeneous group includes:

Gilbert's disease	Probable autosomal dominant
Dubin–Johnson syndrome	Variable autosomal dominant
Defective bilirubin conjugation	
Crigler–Najjar or Arias Type 1	Autosomal recessive
Arias Type 2	Autosomal dominant
Benign recurrent cholestasis	Autosomal recessive
Fatal progressive cholestasis	
(Byler's disease)	Autosomal recessive

Biliary Atresia
This may occur in chromosomal trisomies or be the result of intrauterine viral hepatitis. Most cases are of unknown cause, and recurrence seems rare in sibs regardless of cause, though no satisfactory figures exist.

Polycystic Disease of the Liver and Congenital Hepatic Fibrosis
A variety of forms can be recognized pathologically, depending on the predominance of fibrosis or cystic change, and the degree of renal involvement (*see* Chapter 18). All appear to follow autosomal recessive inheritance. Adult polycystic kidney disease (autosomal dominant) rarely has more than a few hepatic cysts. It is doubtful whether a separate entity of polycystic liver disease without renal involvement exists.

Adult Chronic Liver Disease
In patients with an autoimmune cause, a strong association with other autoimmune disorders and the presence of various autoantibodies, suggests the action of a dominant gene affecting immune responses. A few striking familial aggregations of cirrhosis and hepatoma have been found to result from hepatitis virus, and to have been maternally transmitted[33]. Susceptibility to persistence of hepatitis virus may itself follow autosomal recessive inheritance.

References
1. David T. J. and O'Callaghan S. E. (1975) Oesophageal atresia in the South-West of England. *J. Med. Genet.* **12**, 1–11.
2. Mosbech J. and Videbaek A. (1955) On the etiology of esophageal carcinoma. *J. Natl Cancer Inst.* **15**, 1665–1673.
3. Kmet J. and Mahboubi E. (1972) Oesophageal cancer in the Caspian littoral of Iran: initial studies. *Science* **175**, 846–853.
4. Howel-Evans W., Clarke C. A. and Sheppard P. M. (1958) Carcinoma of oesophagus with keratosis palmaris et plantaris (tylosis). A study of two families. *Q. J. Med.* **17**, 413–429.

5. Harper P. S., Harper R. M. J. and Howel-Evans W. (1970) Carcinoma of the oesophagus with tylosis. *Q. J. Med.* **39**, 317–333.
6. Daentl D. L. and Passarge E. (1972) Familial agenesis of the diaphragm. *Birth Defects* **8**, No. 2. 24–26.
7. David T. J. and Illingworth C. A. (1976) Diaphragmatic hernia in the South-West of England. *J. Med. Genet.* **13**, 253–262.
8. Carter C. O. and Evans K. A. (1969) Inheritance of congenital pyloric stenosis. *J. Med. Genet.* **6**, 233–254.
9. Dodge J. (1973) Genetics of hypertrophic pyloric stenosis. *Clin. Gastroenterol.* **2**, No. 3, 523–538.
10. Lubinsky M., Herrmann J., Kosseff A. L. et al. (1974) Autosomal dominant sex-dependent transmission of the Wiedemann-Beckwith syndrome. *Lancet* **1**, 932.
11. Czeisl P. (1980) Recurrence risk of omphalocele. *Lancet* **2**, 470.
12. Osuna A. and Lindham S. (1976) Four cases of omphalocele in two generations of the same family. *Clin. Genet.* **9**, 354–356.
13. Blyth H. M. and Dickson J. A. S. (1969) Apple peel syndrome (congenital intestinal atresia). *J. Med. Genet.* **6**, 275–277.
14. McConnell R. B. (1966) *The Genetics of Gastrointestinal Disorders.* London, Oxford University Press.
15. Cowan W. K. (1973) Genetics of duodenal and gastric ulcer. *Clin. Gastroenterol.* **2**, 539–546.
16. Ashley D. J. B. (1969) Gastric cancer in Wales. *J. Med. Genet.* **6**, 76–79.
17. Harper P. S. (1973) Heredity and gastrointestinal tumours. *Clin. Gastroenterol.* **2**, 675–701.
18. Varis K. (1971) A family study of chronic gastritis: histological, immunological and functional aspects. *Scand. J. Gastroenterol.* **6**, Suppl. 13, 1–50.
19. Velde K. te, Abels J., Anders G. et al. (1964) A family study of pernicious anaemia by an immunological method. *J. Lab. Clin. Med.* **64**, 176–187.
20. David T. J. and Ajdukiewicz A. B. (1975) A family study of coeliac disease. *J. Med. Genet.* **12**, 79–82.
21. Macdonald W. C., Dobbins W. O. and Rubin C. E. (1965) Studies of the familial nature of celiac sprue using biopsy of the small intestine. *N. Engl. J. Med.* **272**, 448–456.
22. Stokes P. L., Asquith P. and Cooke W. T. (1973) Genetics of coeliac disease. *Clin. Gastroenterol.* **2**, 547–556.
23. Dennis N. R. and Stokes C. R. (1978) Risk of coeliac disease in children of patients and effect of HLA genotype. *J. Med. Genet.* **15**, 20–22.
24. Macmahon B. (1955) Data on the etiology of acute intussusception in childhood. *Am. J. Hum. Genet.* **7**, 430–438.
25. Kirsner J. B. (1973) Genetic aspects of inflammatory bowel disease. *Clin. Gastroenterol.* **2**, 557–575.
26. Fried K. and Vure E. (1974) A lethal autosomal recessive enterocolitis of early infancy. *Clin. Genet.* **6**, 195–196.
27. Pierce E. R. (1968) Some genetic aspects of familial polyposis of the colon in a kindred of 1422 members. *Dis. Colon Rectum* **11**, 321–329.
28. Passarge E. (1972) Genetic heterogeneity and recurrence risk of congenital intestinal aganglionosis. *Birth Defects* **8**, No. 2, 63–67.
29. Gerald P. S., Davis C., Say B. et al. (1972) Syndromal associations of imperforate anus: the cat eye syndrome. *Birth Defects* **8**, No. 2, 79–84.
30. Sibert J. R. (1978) Hereditary pancreatitis in England and Wales. *J. Med. Genet.* **15**, 189–201.
31. Saddi R. and Feingold J. (1974) Idiopathic haemochromatosis: an autosomal recessive disease. *Clin. Genet.* **5**, 234–241.

32. Simon M., Bourel M. and Genetet B. (1977) Idiopathic haemochromatosis. Demonstration of recessive transmission and early detection by family HLA typing. *N. Engl. J. Med.* **297,** 1017–1021.
33. Ohbayashi A., Okochi K. and Mayumi M. (1972) Familial clustering of asymptomatic carriers of Australia antigen and patients with chronic liver disease or primary liver cancer. *Gastroenterology* **62,** 618–625.
34. Warren J., Evans K. and Carter C. O. (1980) Offspring of patients with tracheo-oesophageal fistula. *J. Med. Genet.* **16,** 338.

Further Reading

Bergsma D. (1972) Gastrointestinal tract including liver and pancreas. In: *The Clinical Delineation of Birth Defects. Part 13.* Baltimore, Williams & Wilkins.
McConnell R. B. (1966) *The Genetics of Gastrointestinal Disorders.* London, Oxford University Press.
McConnell R. B. (ed.) (1973) Genetics of gastrointestinal disorders. *Clin. Gastroenterol.* **2,** No. 3.

CHAPTER EIGHTEEN

Renal Disease

Polycystic Kidney Disease

Renal cystic disease may occur in a number of generalized syndromes, notably in trisomy 13 and 18, tuberous sclerosis, Meckel's syndrome and cerebrohepatorenal syndrome (autosomal recessive); it may also be secondary to chronic obstruction or recurrent infection and there is considerable argument over classification among pathologists. Thus the question to be asked is not just whether the case is one of renal cystic disease, but to what is this due? Once the various other causes have been excluded (not always an easy task) primary polycystic disease falls into two distinct groups:

    1. Adult polycystic disease, following autosomal dominant inheritance.

    2. Infantile polycystic disease, heterogeneous but following autosomal recessive inheritance.

Adult Polycystic Disease

Onset is commonly in early adult life, but is extremely variable; an affected child of 3 years has been recorded[1], while mild cases may be found incidentally at autopsy in old age. Counselling of young, apparently healthy family members presents problems since there are no satisfactory data on the age at which presence of the gene can be excluded. All such individuals should have a careful examination, urinalaysis and pyelography; ultrasound and CT scan may prove useful aids (*see* p. 225).

    Apparently isolated cases should not be accepted as new mutations unless both parents are alive and have been shown to be normal.

Infantile Polycystic Disease

This has been subdivided into four types on the basis of age of onset and pathological appearance[2].

    a. Perinatal. Huge kidneys at birth; rapidly fatal.

    b. Neonatal. Onset in first month of life; usually fatal by three months.

    c. Infantile. Onset in first 6 months; liver prominently involved also.

    d. Juvenile. Onset 1—5 years. Severe liver involvement.

    All follow autosomal recessive inheritance. The splitting has some value since each type appears to be constant within a family. The histology is distinct from that of adult polycystic disease; thus it is vital for an accurate autopsy to be done on the proband to avoid confusion with this form and to exclude non-Mendelian causes. Where such information is not available, particularly in isolated cases with onset after the neonatal period, both parents should be studied to exclude an asymptomatic case of the dominantly inherited form. Prenatal diagnosis by ultrasonography is now feasible in the most severe types.

Medullary Cystic Disease (juvenile nephronophthisis; microcystic disease) This disorder, probably the commonest cause of childhood renal failure after infection, with incidence around 1 in 50 000, generally follows autosomal recessive inheritance. The mean age at onset is 9 years, and of death 16 years. Syndromal associations, notably with retinitis pigmentosa and cerebral degeneration have been described and appear to follow the same mode of inheritance.

A dominantly inherited form has been documented in a few families with a rapidly progressive course[3]. Onset is in adult life (mean 29 years) so there should be no risk of confusion with the childhood form. Both types should be distinguished from the benign *medullary sponge kidney,* where no clear familial tendency has been shown.

Hereditary Nephropathies

a. Congenital nephrosis. This is a heterogeneous group. In the rare Finnish type (autosomal recessive), prenatal diagnosis is feasible from a greatly raised amniotic fluid alphafetoprotein[4] (presumably derived from fetal urine). The more recently recognized focal medullary glomerulosclerosis is more variable in clinical presentation and course, but is also probably autosomal recessive.

b. Idiopathic (minimal change) childhood nephrotic syndrome. A careful family study has shown a 6 per cent risk to sibs[5].

c. Amyloidosis. Renal involvement may occur in association with some of the primary amyloid neuropathies and with familial Mediterranean fever (autosomal dominant).

d. Alport's syndrome (hereditary nephropathy with nerve deafness). The mode of inheritance is disputed. Male-to-male transmission is reduced and females are often mildly affected. Heterogeneity is likely. Autosomal dominant inheritance is probable in some families, with reduced penetrance when transmitted by males. Others may be truly X-linked, with carrier females usually showing a degree of haematuria[6]. Individual families should be carefully evaluated to see which mode appears to be operating.

e. Other inherited nephropathies. A number of unusual forms have been reported, usually autosomal dominant in inheritance.

Urinary Tract Malformations

a. Renal agenesis. The recurrence risk in sibs is low (3 per cent) for bilateral agenesis[7]. The same risk is probable for unilateral agenesis (though many cases are undetected).

b. Hydronephrosis. Most bilateral cases are secondary to obstruction or other disorders. Unilateral hydronephrosis following autosomal dominant inheritance has been recorded.

c. Bladder exstrophy. Recurrence in sibs is very rare (1 of 162 sibs in the only series available)[8]. Prenatal diagnosis from raised amniotic fluid alphafetoprotein or fetoscopy might be feasible, but seems unwise (especially the latter) in view of the low risk of recurrence.

d. 'Prune belly' syndrome (abdominal muscle deficiency, megaureter, megacystis, undescended testis). Almost all cases are male. Recurrence in sibs is rare (less than 1 per cent) and several discordant monozygotic twin pairs are known.

e. Urethral valves. Satisfactory risk figures are not available, but the risk is certainly small in sibs.

f. Hypospadias (incidence 1 in 3000 males). The recurrence risk in male sibs is around 10 per cent, and in children of affected males, the risk is similar. The risk for offspring of female sibs of patients is uncertain. Care must be taken to distinguish various intersexual states and Mendelian syndromes (such as the Smith—Lemli—Opitz syndrome).

Vesico-ureteric Reflux
A family study[9] has shown a risk of around 10 per cent to sibs (about 10 X the population frequency) which is relevant to the early detection and prevention of renal scarring. A similar proportion of parents were affected.

Renal Stones
Cystinuria (Chapter 20) is autosomal recessive in inheritance, so sibs of affected children deserve careful screening for this relatively common (about 1 in 7000) and readily treatable disorder. Urate stones may reflect an underlying hyperuricaemia, but often do not. The common calcium-containing stones resulting from hypercalciuria have not so far been shown to have any clear genetic basis, though it would not be surprising were this to be so.

Table 18.1. Renal transport defects

Cystinuria Renal glycosuria Hartnup's disease Dibasic aminoaciduria Fanconi's syndrome (usually secondary to cystinosis)	Autosomal recessive
Lowe's syndrome Familial hypophosphataemia Nephrogenic diabetes insipidus	X-linked (variable female expression)
Renal tubular acidosis	Autosomal dominant (when familial)

Renal Transport Disorders

Table 18.1 lists some of these. As expected with inborn errors of metabolism, most are autosomal recessive, but the three X-linked conditions are all variable in the heterozygous female; most carriers of Lowe's (oculocerebrorenal) syndrome are detectable by lens opacities, while heterozygotes for familial hypophosphataemia may be short and have low phosphate serum levels. Renal tubular acidosis is heterogeneous; many cases are sporadic, but numerous families with autosomal dominant inheritance exist, and urine acidification in the parents should be checked before giving a low risk for a subsequent affected child.

Results are now available of a large study of adult polycystic kidney disease showing that either pyelography with tomograms or radionuclide imaging will detect almost all gene caries over 19 years old, the risk of carrying the gene being under 5 per cent for those normal by these tests[10].

References

1. Carter C. O. (1974) Polycystic disease presenting in childhood. In: Bergsma D. (ed.), *Birth Defects – Urinary System and Others.* Vol. 10, No. 4, pt 16. Baltimore, Williams & Wilkins, pp. 16–21.
2. Blyth H. and Ockenden B. G. (1971) Polycystic disease of kidneys and liver presenting in childhood. *J. Med. Genet.* 8, 257–284.
3. Gardner K. D. (1974) Cystic diseases of the kidney: a perspective on medullary cystic disease. In: Bergsma D. (ed.), *Birth Defects – Urinary System and Others.* Vol. 10, No. 4, pt 16, pp. 29–31.
4. Seppala M., Rapola J., Huttunen N. P. et al. (1976) Congenital nephrotic syndrome: prenatal diagnosis and genetic counselling by estimation of amniotic-fluid and maternal serum alpha-fetoprotein. *Lancet* 2, 123–124.
5. Bader P. I., Grove J., Nance W. E. et al. (1974) Inheritance of idiopathic nephrotic syndrome. In: Bergsma D. (ed.), *Birth Defects – Urinary System and Others.* Vol. 10, No. 4, pt 16, pp. 73–79.
6. O'Neill W. M., Atkins C. L. and Bloomer H. A. (1978) Hereditary nephritis: a reexamination of its clinical and genetic features. *Ann. Intern. Med.* 88, 176–182.
7. Carter C. O., Evans K. and Pescia G. (1979) A family study of renal agenesis. *J. Med. Genet.* 16, 176–188.
8. Ives E., Coffey R. and Carter C. O. (1980) *J. Med. Genet.* 17, 139–141.
9. De Vargas A., Evans K., Ransley P. et al. (1978) A family study of vesicoureteric reflux. *J. Med. Genet.* 15, 85–96.
10. Milutinovic J., Fialkow P. J., Phillips L. A. et al. (1980) Autosomal dominant polycystic kidney disease: early diagnosis and data for genetic counselling. *Lancet* 1, 1203–1206.

Further Reading

Bergsma D. (ed.) (1974) *Birth Defects – Urinary System and Others.* Vol. 10, No. 4, pt 16. Baltimore, Williams & Wilkins.
Gardner K. D. (ed.) (1976) *Cystic Diseases of the Kidney.* New York, Wiley.

CHAPTER NINETEEN

Endocrine Disorders

Diabetes Mellitus

Despite the high prevalence of diabetes and the widespread knowledge that hereditary factors are involved, very few patients with diabetes, in the author's experience, attend a genetic counselling clinic. This is perhaps fortunate in view of the confusion that exists over the genetic risks! Considering the large amount of work undertaken, the disparity in results is truly amazing. A good review of the subject has recently been produced[1], though the practical data for counselling are scanty. In it Neel admits that his view of diabetes as 'a geneticist's nightmare' ten years previously has not changed significantly.

Many of the problems in estimating genetic risks in diabetes arise from the obvious heterogeneity of the disorder and only recently has evidence emerged to help separate some of the major categories. It is likely that the overall risk figures represent a mixture of a large group where the risks are extremely low with some smaller groups where there is a high recurrence risk. The following groups can be provisionally distinguished:

1. Insulin-dependent diabetes
    a. Associated with persistent islet cell antibodies and with autoantibodies to other endocrine glands, especially adrenal. (Around 5 per cent of all insulin-dependent diabetes.)
    b. Possibly virally induced, not associated with other endocrine disorders and probably with little recurrence risk.
2. Non-insulin-dependent diabetes
    a. Maturity onset. Common.
    b. Juvenile type. Rare; follows autosomal dominant pattern.
3. Diabetes associated with other primary genetic disorders.

Apart from group 3 and the rare juvenile form (*2b*) showing autosomal dominant inheritance, no theoretical prediction of risks is possible and empiric risk estimates are widely divergent. *Table* 19.1 summarizes the available data. The different series are discussed by Simpson (in Creutzfeldt et al.[1]; Simpson's own study[2] is one of the most thorough. It is to be hoped that it will soon be possible to completely revise these estimates in the light of a more logical classification of the different forms. In the face of such extreme variations in risk, it is difficult to know what figures to give to patients. The author's practice is first to warn families of

Table 19.1. The range of genetic risks in diabetes (after Rimoin and Schimke, 1971)

Family member(s) affected	Individual at risk	Risk estimates (%)	
		Clinical diabetes	Abnormal GTT
One parent	Child	4–10	
Both parents	Child	3–37.5	6–56
Sib	Sib	2.4–11.7	18–39
Monozygotic twin	Co-twin	10–97	14–100
Dizygotic twin	Co-twin	3–37	9–39

the inadequacy of our knowledge, secondly to stress that there are different types of diabetes, some with a small genetic component, others with a larger, and thirdly to give risks only for overt clinical diabetes, ignoring the estimates for abnormal glucose tolerance tests. For insulin-dependent juvenile type diabetes, a risk of diabetes in the first 20 years of life of 3 per cent for children of an affected parent is given; a similar risk is given for a further child with diabetes being born to healthy parents with one diabetic child. A risk for children of conjugal diabetics of around 20 per cent for clinical diabetes in the first 20 years of life is given, and around 50 per cent of diabetes developing at some stage of life.

For non-insulin-dependent 'maturity type' diabetes, the ultimate risks are likely to be higher, around 10 per cent for first-degree relatives, but this is of less significance since the majority of patients will be mildly affected relatively late in life.

The question of whether diabetics should marry each other and have children requires mention, if only because a World Health Organization Commission dogmatically (and unwisely) advised that they should not, on eugenic grounds. It is clear that the risk of diabetes in the children of such couples is considerably increased, and possibly also the severity; there may, therefore, be good grounds for such couples avoiding childbearing or limiting their family. The eugenic grounds for doing so are far from secure, however, as emphasized by Edwards[3]. The main population effect is probably a rearrangement of the diabetic children being born, to give more to diabetic parents and less to non-diabetic, with no clear rise in frequency of the disease and probably a decrease if the diabetic couples have small families. A final reason for caution regarding the eugenic aspects is that, as Neel mentions, with declining food sources man may need the 'thrifty genotype' of the diabetic in the future.

The risk of developing diabetes is not the only factor to be considered in giving genetic counselling to diabetic families. The offspring of a diabetic mother face special hazards, though these appear to be declining markedly with better diabetic control during pregnancy. The perinatal mortality has been shown to correlate with the severity of maternal diabetes; one large study has given an overall perinatal mortality of 20 per cent, rising to almost 40 per cent in the most severe group[4]. Although risks have declined since these data were collected, they are far from negligible.

There is also an increase in the incidence of congenital malformations in the offspring of the diabetic mother, with a threefold excess over the general population. Petersen et al.[5] showed a 6·4 per cent incidence compared with 2·1 per cent in a control population. When subdivided by presence of vascular complications in the mother, the malformation rate was 10·7 per cent in the offspring of those with vascular complications, 4·4 per cent in those without. It is likely, but not certain that these risks are also declining with improved diabetic control.

A few rare specific malformations seem to occur particularly in the offspring of diabetic mothers, including sacral agenesis, proximal femoral deficiency, and related 'caudal regression syndromes'. The recurrence risk of these is small in relation to the other malformations, which do not follow any specific pattern.

Table 19.2. Endocrine deficiency disorders

Congenital absence of pituitary	Probable autosomal recessive
Familial panhypopituitarism	Autosomal recessive or X-linked recessive
Isolated growth hormone deficiency	Autosomal recessive or autosomal dominant
Laron type pituitary dwarfism	Autosomal recessive
Isolated TSH deficiency	Usually sporadic
Isolated HGH deficiency	Usually sporadic
Isolated gonadotrophin deficiency	Autosomal recessive
Diabetes insipidus – hereditary vasopressin deficient	Autosomal dominant; rarely X-linked recessive
Diabetes insipidus – nephrogenic	X-linked (intermediate in females)
Hypoparathyroidism (idiopathic)	Usually sporadic. Rarely X-linked recessive
Hypoparathyroidism with adrenal failure and moniliasis	Autosomal recessive
Pseudohypoparathyroidism (Albright's hereditary osteodystrophy)	Usually X-linked dominant. Possibly autosomal dominant in a few families
Congenital hypothyroidism, goitrous	Autosomal recessive *see* p. 229
Congenital hypothyroidism, agoitrous	*see* p. 229
Adrenal cortical hypoplasia	Usually sporadic. Rarely X-linked recessive
Adrenal cortical hypoplasia with cerebral sclerosis	X-linked recessive

Endocrine Deficiency Disorders

A large number of these conditions exists, of which some represent primary inborn errors of metabolism (usually recessively inherited), while others represent failures of development of the particular organ (usually sporadic). An increasingly recognized group is that characterized by autoantibodies against a variety of endocrine glands. *Table* 19.2 summarizes some of these primary deficiency states, along with what is known of their inheritance.

Endocrine deficiencies of adult life, including hypothyroidism, Addison's disease and hypopituitarism, rarely carry a high recurrence risk within a family unless associated with autoimmunity. In such a situation, there is an increased risk not only of the disorder affecting the propositus, but of autoimmune disease of other endocrine glands, including diabetes, as well as of disorders such as pernicious anaemia. High titres of autoantibodies may be found in relatives in the absence of clinical disease and it is likely that in many families the general predisposition to autoimmunity follows autosomal dominant inheritance. Unfortunately, no accurate figures exist for the risk of clinical endocrine problems in relatives, but it is certainly wise for the presence of autoantibodies to be checked in first-degree relatives when the endocrine failure in the propositus is found to be autoimmune in origin.

Congenital Hypothyroidism

Most cases are due to failure of thyroid gland development and are sporadic; occasional occurrence in sibs may indicate recessively inherited forms which cannot at present be distinguished. It is likely that systematic newborn screening[6] will clarify the recurrence risks.

The presence of a goitre in a non-endemic region indicates that an inborn error of thyroxine synthesis is likely; the various types all follow autosomal recessive inheritance, including Pendred's syndrome, where defective iodine organification is associated with nerve deafness.

Absence of thyroxine-binding globulins may be X-linked recessive or autosomal dominant; it is usually harmless, but may be confused with hypothyroidism biochemically.

Endocrine Overproduction Disorders

These are rarely familial, except for thyrotoxicosis, where the risk to sibs is around 1 in 6 for females (considerably less for males). The recognition of an autoimmune basis for most cases should prompt a careful search for clinical or immunological evidence of other types of autoimmune endocrine disease in close relatives. There is a close association between Graves' disease and the HLA antigens DW3 and B8.

Occasional families with isolated hyperparathyroidism following autosomal dominant inheritance have been reported, but most cases are sporadic, as are most instances of Cushing's syndrome and of pituitary tumours, unless forming part of multiple endocrine adenomatosis, described below.

Multiple Endocrine Adenomatosis [7]

Type 1. Parathyroid, pituitary and pancreatic endocrine tumours are most frequent. Inheritance is autosomal dominant.

Type 2. This is heterogeneous. Medullary carcinoma of the thyroid may occur alone or coexist with phaeochromocytoma and with mucosal neuromas.

Some patients may be 'Marfanoid' in appearance. Inheritance is usually autosomal dominant.

Both major forms are important examples of high-risk neoplastic disorders, where recognition of the Mendelian inheritance can prevent fatal disease in relatives, quite apart from the importance of genetic counselling.

Congenital Adrenal Hyperplasia (Adrenogenital Syndrome)
At least 8 types exist, resulting from different disorders of steroid hormone biosynthesis; all follow autosomal recessive inheritance. The most important type, 21-hydroxylase deficiency, is closely linked to the HLA system[8], allowing prediction of recurrence in a family and possibly prenatal prediction when reliable HLA typing of amniotic cells becomes feasible. Direct prenatal diagnosis from amniotic fluid also appears possible [9], and may allow early treatment to avoid a salt-losing crisis. It is debatable whether termination of an affected pregnancy will often be requested in view of the good results of early treatment.

Hypogonadism

Numerous types exist in each sex; they may be isolated defects or be part of more generalized syndromes. The accompanying infertility militates against a clear inheritance pattern in many cases, and a specific clinical

Table 19.3. Some major genetic causes of hypogonadism and allied states

Type	*Inheritance*
Male	
Klinefelter's syndrome (XXY)	Usually sporadic
Kallman's syndrome (hypogonadotrophic hypogonadism with anosmia)	X-linked recessive
Reifenstein's syndrome (hypogonadism with hypospadias)	X-linked recessive
Prader–Willi syndrome (hypogonadism with obesity, hypotonia, mental retardation, small hands and feet)	Usually sporadic (risk to sibs under 3%)
Female	
Turner's syndrome (XO)	Usually sporadic
XX gonadal dysgenesis	Autosomal recessive (sex linked)
XY gonadal dysgenesis	X-linked recessive (probably)
Testicular feminization	X-linked recessive

cytogenetic and endocrine diagnosis is critical. Since many cases will not be recognized until puberty and will in any case not be able to reproduce, counselling is most commonly needed for the healthy sibs. The risk for their offspring will be extremely low except for the sisters of patients with X-linked disorders, such as the Kallmann and Reifenstein syndromes, and testicular feminization. Since these disorders are effectively 'lethal' in genetic terms, a third of cases will probably represent new mutations, so that the risk of mothers of an isolated case being a carrier will be 2/3, and for the sisters of such a case, 1/3. This will give a risk of 1/3 and 1/6 for the sons (or XY offspring) of mothers and sisters respectively.

A few of the major forms of hypogonadism are summarized in *Table 19.3*. Rimoin and Schimke give an excellent account of the various syndromes.

Infertility

Genetic counselling in cases of infertility may seem a contradiction in terms, since the problem is only discovered when a couple is actively trying to conceive. However, two important questions which need to be asked (but frequently are not) by those attempting to investigate and treat infertility are:

1. Is the infertility one aspect of a genetic disorder that might be transmitted?

2. Will correction of infertility give an increased risk of malformations in the offspring?

The genetic causes of infertility are numerous and in part overlap with those of hypogonadism already mentioned, and as with these, it is only X-linked or autosomal recessive disorders that are of practical importance for counselling, since only in these will unaffected people be at risk of having an affected child.

Disorders of sperm production include abnormalities of chromosome pairing in meiosis, cilial defects affecting motility and a variety of poorly defined biochemical disorders. Primary sex chromosome disorders include XXY (Klinefelter) and XO (Turner) syndromes. Mendelian disorders causing relative infertility include myotonic dystrophy.

The question of increased risk to offspring arises principally in those patients in whom apparent infertility is really a reflection of early unrecognized fetal loss as a result of abnormal gamete production. The most important group to detect is where one parent carries a balanced translocation, where the risk of an unbalanced chromosome abnormality in a pregnancy that goes to term is considerable, especially where the defect is carried by a female. This problem is closely related to that of recurrent abortion, considered below.

Genetic Counselling and Recurrent Abortions

Most women with a history of recurrent abortions will be under the care of a gynaecologist, who will have already searched for a gynaecological cause and will have excluded most serious maternal disorders. A genetic basis is usually considered if:

a. There is evidence of abnormality in an abortus.

   b. Chromosome studies of mother or abortus have shown an abnormality.

   c. There is a family history of some disease that might be relevant.

The main question to be answered is not so much whether or not another abortion will occur, but what is the risk that a pregnancy reaching term will result in an abnormality? The question of amniocentesis may also arise: clearly one does not want to expose a pregnancy to any added risk of abortion unless there is a likelihood of an abnormality detectable by this.

There will be many women where careful search reveals no genetic or other factors involved, but with care considerable help can be given by the following measures:

   1. Examination of the abortus where possible — this may identify major abnormalities such as neural tube defects.

   2. Cytogenetic study of the abortus — as discussed in Chapter 4, chromosomal abnormalities are an exceedingly common cause.

   3. Cytogenetic study of parents. This is especially important where a translocation is a possibility and should always be done where the abortus is known to be chromosomally abnormal.

   4. Search for possible lethal Mendelian causes, e.g. consanguinity, increasing the risk of autosomal recessive lethals, X-linked dominant disorders lethal in the male, myotonic dystrophy giving heavy fetal loss in the offspring of mildly affected women.

The most important group to detect are the autosomal translocations, where one parent is a balanced translocation carrier. As stated in Chapter 4, these carry a significant risk of an abnormal liveborn offspring, probably around 12 per cent where the carrier is female, but nearer 5 per cent where the male is the carrier. Amniocentesis is clearly indicated in any such pregnancy, and there is no evidence that it is accompanied by a greater risk of abortion in such a situation.

It is important for couples to realize that spontaneous abortion is an exceedingly common event, occurring in at least 1 in 8 *recognized* pregnancies. Thus 1 in 64 women might be expected to have two consecutive abortions on grounds of chance alone, and unless there are other reasons, it is probably not worth investigating women unless they have had at least three spontaneous abortions.

References

1. Creutzfeldt W., Kobberling J. and Neel J. V. (ed.) (1976) *The Genetics of Diabetes Mellitus,* Berlin, Springer.
2. Simpson N. E. (1968) Diabetes in the families of diabetics. *Canad. Med. Assoc. J.* **98,** 427–432.
3. Edwards J. H. (1969) Should diabetics marry? *Lancet* **1,** 1045–1047.
4. Gellis S. S. and Hsia D. Y. (1959) Perinatal mortality in offspring of diabetic mothers. *Am. J. Dis. Child.* **97,** 1–41.
5. Pedersen L. M., Tygstrup I. and Pedersen J. (1964) Congenital malformations in newborn infants of diabetic women. *Lancet* **1,** 1124–1126.

6. Neonatal Screening for Congenital Hypothyroidism in Europe. Report of the Newborn Committee of the European Thyroid Association (1979) *Acta Endocrinol. (Kbh)* **90,** Suppl. 223, 1–29.
7. Schimke R. N. (1978) *Genetics and Cancer in Man.* London, Churchill-Livingstone, pp. 47–54.
8. Dupont B., Smithwick E. M., Oberfield S. E. et al. (1977) Close genetic linkage between HLA and congenital adrenal hyperplasia (21-hydroxylase deficiency). *Lancet* **2,** 1309–1312.
9. Hughes I. A. and Laurence K. M. (1979) Antenatal diagnosis of congenital adrenal hyperplasia. *Lancet* **2,** 7–9.

Further Reading
Rimoin D. L. and Schimke R. N. (1971) *Genetic Disorders of the Endocrine Glands.* St Louis, Mosby.

CHAPTER TWENTY

Inborn Errors of Metabolism

It seems likely that most, if not all, Mendelian disorders will eventually prove to fall into this category, being the result of a deficient or defective specific gene product. For practical purposes it seems wise to restrict the term to those conditions where some form of metabolic basis has been clearly identified, but each year more diseases are added to the group. In many cases, the discovery of a specific metabolic basis radically changes the concept of a disease; thus, Tay—Sachs disease is no longer thought of as purely a brain degeneration, but as a generalized metabolic disorder, and the preventive measures of carrier detection and prenatal diagnosis involve biochemical and genetic techniques far removed from those generally associated with neurology. Xeroderma pigmentosum and allied disorders of DNA repair are further examples of disorders entering the inborn error category, and the muscular dystrophies seem likely to join them in the near future.

From the viewpoint of genetic counselling, inborn errors of metabolism have several characteristics which must be taken into account.

1. Almost all follow Mendelian recessive inheritance, the great majority being autosomal.

2. Precise biochemical techniques for early recognition, carrier detection and prenatal diagnosis are often available.

3. Genetic heterogeneity is frequent, but can usually be detected biochemically if not clinically. Further splitting of apparently well-defined disorders will undoubtedly continue.

No attempt is made here to describe or even list the large number of inborn errors, mostly very rare, that have been documented, and if a disorder is not mentioned it can be assumed that the inheritance is autosomal recessive. This means that unless consanguinity exists, or the gene is especially common in a particular population, the risks to the offspring of healthy sibs or more distant relatives is extremely low, and that carrier detection or prenatal diagnosis is not likely to be required. Indeed such relatives will often need active dissuasion from tests whose margin of error may be considerably greater than the individual's prior risk of having an affected child.

Tables 20.1 and 20.2 give those disorders known to follow X-linked or autosomal dominant inheritance. The X-linked group is especially important for carrier detection, since the female carrier will have a 50 per cent risk of transmitting the condition to her sons (*see* Chapter 5). Those disorders for which prenatal diagnosis is feasible have been listed in *Table 6.7*, p. 88, and further discussion of the role of prenatal diagnosis for

Table 20.1. X-linked inborn errors of metabolism

Disorder	*Enzyme defect* (where relevant)
Agammaglobulinaemia, Bruton type (also some families with Swiss type)	
Angiokeratoma (Fabry's disease)	α-galactosidase
Glucose-6-phosphate dehydrogenase deficiency	G6PD
Granulomatous disease	NADPH oxidase
Glycogenosis Type VIII	Liver phosphorylase kinase
Haemophilia A	Factor VIII (procoagulant subunit)
Haemophilia B	Factor IX
Hyperammonaemia Type I	Ornithine carbamyl transferase
Hypophosphataemic rickets	Renal tubule phosphate transport defect
Ichthyosis, X-linked	Steroid sulphatase
Lesch–Nyhan syndrome	HGPRTase
Menkes' syndrome	Defective copper absorption
Mucopolysaccharidosis II (Hunter's syndrome)	Iduronate sulphatase

See Table 2.3, p. 37, for a fuller list of X-linked disorders.

Table 20.2. Inborn errors of metabolism following autosomal dominant inheritance

Porphyrias {	Acute intermittent Variegate Coproporphyria Protoporphyria
Type II hyperlipidaemia (rarely homozygous)	
Hereditary angioedema	

inherited metabolic disease is also given in Chapter 6. The recent development of techniques of fetal blood sampling is likely to extend this list greatly in the near future.

Some of the disorders listed in the tables are discussed in more detail in other chapters, e.g. haemophilia and haemoglobinopathies (Chapter 21). The following notes deal with some of the situations particularly relevant to genetic counselling in individual conditions.

Phenylketonuria

With a mean frequency of around 1 in 10 000 births in Britain (carrier frequency 1 in 50), this is one of the commoner inborn errors. Successful dietary treatment and newborn screening has largely transferred the burden of genetic counselling onto the daughters of the next generation. Here, although the risk of transmitting phenylketonuria is low (around 1 per cent) there is a high risk of brain damage in *all* offspring of affected women due to phenylalanine crossing the placenta. It is not yet clear whether strict dietary treatment in pregnancy averts this. There is no evidence that such problems occur among the offspring of asymptomatic individuals with moderately raised blood phenylalanine detected by screening.

Prenatal diagnosis is not feasible except for the very rare and usually fatal form, due to dihydropteridine reductase deficiency, which does not respond to usual dietary treatment. In the classic form due to phenylalanine hydroxylase deficiency the enzyme is confined to the liver. Carrier detection is feasible (Chapter 5) but not often required.

Histidinaemia
Most cases appear to be asymptomatic and the original association thought to exist with speech problems and mental retardation seems doubtful. There is no evidence of a significant maternal effect in the heterozygous offspring of affected women.

Cystinuria
Renal calculi are the only significant clinical feature; heterozygotes in one of the two forms may excrete small amounts of amino acids in the urine, but are symptomless and must not be confused with the affected homozygotes, where large quantities of cystine and other dibasic amino acids are excreted. The disorder is quite distinct from *cystinosis* (also autosomal recessive) which is a generalized storage disease of cystine, with much more serious clinical effects, including renal failure.

Galactosaemia
Recognition of this rapidly fatal disorder is important not only because effective treatment exists, but to allow immediate diagnosis from cord blood in a subsequent pregnancy. Distinction of classic galactosaemia must also be made from the form due to galactokinase deficiency in which cataract is the only abnormality, and from harmless enzyme variants that may be picked up by screening programmes. Prenatal diagnosis by amniocentesis is feasible and has also been reported using fetal blood sampling. Such procedures seem of doubtful justification since treatment is effective and prenatal damage of the infant by the disease exceptional. Employing such techniques just because they are technically feasible is inexcusable. The various options and their consequences must be frankly discussed with the couple concerned before a decision is made.

Sphingolipidoses

Specific lysosomal enzyme defects have been identified for most disorders in this group, and prenatal diagnosis is feasible in these. Carrier detection is only of significance for Tay—Sachs disease, where the gene is at high frequency in Ashkenazi Jewish populations. Screening for adult carriers, with prenatal diagnosis offered to couples who both carry the gene, has been successfully applied in some American Jewish communities, in which 1 in 30 individuals are carriers. Other important members of the group, all autosomal recessive in inheritance, include Gaucher's, Batten's and Niemann—Pick disease, metachromatic leukodystrophy and generalized gangliosidosis.

Fabry's disease is X-linked, with minor signs, including characteristic skin lesions often detectable in female carriers. The *mucopolysaccharidoses* are mentioned in Chapter 11.

The importance of obtaining a precise enzymatic diagnosis in inborn errors of metabolism has already been stressed, but it is probably more important in the group of lysosomal enzyme deficiencies than any other, since clinical differentiation is often extremely difficult, prognosis poor, but prenatal diagnosis feasible *if* one knows which enzyme is defective (*see* Chapter 6).

Glycogen Storage Diseases

All members of this heterogeneous group are autosomal recessive in inheritance, apart from the exceedingly rare type VIII (X-linked recessive). Type II (Pompe's disease), due to lysosomal acid maltase deficiency, is prenatally diagnosable and exists in two distinct forms, an infantile type with severe cardiomyopathy and cerebral involvement, and a later neuromuscular type that may mimic a muscular dystrophy. The classic type I (Von Gierke) glucose-6-phosphatase deficiency is not prenatally diagnosable, but the milder type III (debrancher deficiency) may be.

Hyperlipidaemias (*see also* Chapter 16)

The classification of these disorders is still in a state of flux. Type I (hyperchylomicronaemia) and type V are autosomal recessive. The relatively common type II (hereditary hypercholesterolaemia), especially important because of its association with early coronary heart disease, is autosomal dominant, with a frequency of around 1 in 400 births in Western populations. Very rare, severely affected homozygotes are well documented. It is most important that this disorder (and other primary hyperlipidaemias) is not diagnosed until it is quite clear that a secondary hyperlipidaemic state due to diabetes, obesity or other factors has been excluded. It is still uncertain whether cord blood lipoproteins will reliably detect the disorder in infants, or whether early treatment modifies the prognosis. It must also be remembered that the prognosis is considerably better in women for whom the risk of early heart disease is considerably less than that of inheriting the gene.

The Porphyrias

The acute porphyrias form the most striking exception to the rule of recessive inheritance for most inborn errors due to enzyme defects. Acute intermittent porphyria, variegate porphyria, hereditary coproporphyria and protoporphyria all follow autosomal dominant inheritance. Careful investigation of urine and faecal porphyrins, and where possible enzyme studies, are needed to exclude subclinical disease. Now that specific enzyme defects are known, prenatal diagnosis may be possible, but seems of doubtful applicability. The severe congenital erythropoietic porphyria follows autosomal recessive inheritance; porphyria cutanea tarda, much the commonest of the group, is usually sporadic, with minimal recurrence risk for family members; it may result from interaction of a relatively common gene with adverse environmental factors such as alcoholic liver damage.

Cholinesterase Deficiency

This important cause of apnoea following muscle relaxation follows autosomal recessive inheritance. Sibs are thus the principal relatives at risk, though since the gene is relatively common it may also be worth testing the parents. Heterozygotes (4 per cent of the population) are not at significant risk of clinical problems and in testing relatives it is most important not to confuse them with affected homozygotes. Since heterozygotes commonly show a moderate reduction in cholinesterase level, the dibucaine number, which measures the degree of inhibition of the enzyme by dibucaine, should be measured. This will be under 25 in affected homozygotes, 50–70 in heterozygotes, and over 75 for normal homozygotes. Other rare genetic variants exist and the subject is clearly discussed by Harris (1975).

Further Reading

Harris H. (ed.) (1975) *The Principles of Human Biochemical Genetics*. Amsterdam, Elsevier.

Kaback M. M. (ed.) (1971) *Tay–Sachs Disease: Screening and Prevention*. New York, Alan Liss.

Scriver C. R. and Rosenberg L. E. (1973) *Amino Acid Metabolism and its Disorders*. Philadelphia, Saunders.

Society for Study of Inborn Errors of Metabolism Reports. Publishers Churchill-Livingstone until 1974; MTP from 1975 onwards.
A valuable annual series of books, each dealing with a specific area of inherited metabolic disease.

Stanbury J. B., Wyngaarden J. B. and Fredrickson D. S. (1978) *The Metabolic Basis of Inherited Disease*. New York, McGraw-Hill.
An invaluable and detailed source book on all aspects of specific inborn errors of metabolism, including those mentioned in this chapter.

CHAPTER TWENTY-ONE

Blood

Disorders of Haemoglobin Structure and Synthesis

This large group, of great importance in many parts of the world, contains perhaps the best understood disorders, in molecular terms, that exist. All are autosomal, most recessive in inheritance, and only a few points will be mentioned here.

Sicke-cell Disease

Sickle-cell disease is exceptionally common in some regions, and the heterozygote frequency approaches 1/8 in some parts of Africa. Thus, carrier testing is of great importance, but fortunately, it is readily feasible using a sickling test screen on the red cells, with haemoglobin electrophoresis as a confirmatory measure. Only couples who are both carriers will be at risk of having an affected child. Heterozygotes are essentially healthy and have partial protection against malaria in endemic areas. It is important for them not to be given the erroneous impression that they have a mild form of the disease.

Prenatal diagnosis using fetal red cells is feasible[1], but has not yet found wide application; development of techniques using amniotic cells may change this (Chapter 6). Screening programmes for carriers have also met with little success, partly because of hasty and ill-judged introduction, partly because of the stigmatization of carriers that has resulted[2].

Numerous other β-chain abnormalities are known, some of which, such as haemoglobin C, may be encountered as genetic compounds with haemoglobin S.

Thalassaemias

Thalassaemias[3], characterized by a failure of globin chain synthesis due to a variety of underlying causes, are another group which is exceedingly common in some regions of the world, as well as in immigrant populations of Europe and America. All are recessively inherited, and various compounds with different abnormal alleles may occur. β-thalassaemia major (Cooley's anaemia) is a major problem in parts of the Mediterranean, the Middle East and Asia, while in South-East Asia forms of α-thalassaemia make a large contribution to intrauterine and neonatal deaths. Carrier detection of most forms is feasible, and prenatal diagnosis from fetal blood is also a real possibility, particularly for β-thalassaemia major, for which there is now considerable experience[4]. The application of genetic engineering techniques to thalassaemias and haemoglobinopathies has been mentioned in Chapter 6, and is especially suitable for types of α-thalassaemia where there is an actual gene deletion.

Hereditary Spherocytosis[5]
This disorder of the red cell membrane follows autosomal dominant inheritance, but haemolysis is often mild, requiring red cell fragility tests to be sure that an individual is not affected. Numerous other causes of spherocytosis must be excluded before this diagnosis is made.

Hereditary Elliptocytosis
Hereditary elliptocytosis is also autosomal dominant. Two forms exist, one of which shows close linkage with the rhesus blood group system.

Glucose-6-Phosphate Dehydrogenase (G6PD) Deficiency
This important red cell enzyme deficiency is particularly common in parts of the Middle East and in people of African descent, but is not unknown in others. Numerous enzyme variants exist, with varying loss of activity which determines severity of disease. The disorder is X-linked recessive, but the gene is so common in some areas (e.g. the Arabian peninsula) that homozygous affected females are frequent. Carrier detection is often feasible, but this depends on the type of the abnormality.

Other Red Cell Enzyme Defects
These are mostly autosomal recessive with the exception of phosphoglycerate kinase deficiency which is X-linked. Some are confined to the red cell, others have generalized clinical effects (e.g. triose phosphate isomerase deficiency). Prenatal diagnosis from fetal blood seems a real possibility for this group, but some can also be detected in cultured amniotic fluid cells.

Pernicious Anaemia
This has already been mentioned in connection with atrophic gastritis (*see* Chapter 17). Congenital vitamin B_{12} deficiency is an exceptionally rare disorder following autosomal recessive inheritance

Rhesus Incompatibility[6]
The prevention of haemolytic disease of the newborn due to rhesus incompatibility has been so successful that there is a danger of overlooking the problem completely. It certainly ranks as one of the major contributions of medical genetics in recent years. Although the genetics of the rhesus system is complex and will not be discussed here, the essential problem arises when a homozygous rhesus-negative woman married to

a rhesus-positive man (heterozygous or homozygous) develops antibodies which will react with the red cells of a rhesus-positive fetus. Sensitization may be the result of a previous pregnancy or abortion, or result from transfusion, and is now usually prevented by giving anti-RhD antibody at the appropriate time.

Once sensitization has occurred, any rhesus-positive fetus will be at risk; this will be 50 per cent of pregnancies where the father is heterozygous, 100 per cent where he is homozygous for the RhD antigen.

Other Blood Group Systems

These are discussed in relation to paternity and zygosity testing in Chapter 7. Most blood group systems do not cause regular clinical problems, though haemolytic disease of the newborn may occur, particularly with the ABO and Kell systems. Most blood group antigens are co-dominant, expressing themselves without interfering with the action of other alleles that may be present.

A variety of disease associations have been described with the ABO blood group system[7], but are too weak to be of use in genetic counselling. Similarly, although blood groups are useful genetic markers in the study of genetic linkage, it is rare to be able to apply this form of information in risk prediction. The linkage between myotonic dystrophy, the secretor locus and the Lutheran blood group is perhaps an exception, but even here its use is limited.

Table 21.1. Hereditary disorders of blood cell production

Blackfan–Diamond red cell hypoplasia	Autosomal recessive
Fanconi's pancytopenia	Autosomal recessive
Infantile hereditary agranulocytosis	Autosomal recessive
Cyclic neutropenia	Autosomal recessive or dominant
Chediak–Higashi syndrome	Autosomal recessive
Chronic granulomatous disease	X-linked recessive (rarely autosomal recessive)
Hereditary isolated thrombocytopenia	X-linked recessive (may be autosomal recessive or autosomal dominant)
Thrombocytopenia with absent radius syndrome	Autosomal recessive
Familial lymphohistiocytosis	Autosomal recessive

White Blood Cells and Platelets

A number of rare genetic disorders exists and information is summarized in *Table* 21.1; there is some overlap with the immune deficiency disorders considered below. A number of syndromal associations with skeletal dysplasias also exist and should be carefully looked for.

Leukaemias are considered in Chapter 22.

Immune Deficiency Diseases[8]

Numerous forms of immune deficiency exist, mostly Mendelian in inheritance and are summarized in *Table* 21.2. The X-linked Bruton type of hypogammaglobulinaemia is particularly important to recognize in view of the high risk to offspring of female carriers. Some carrier women can be recognized by lowered immunoglobulin levels in their blood. The proportion that *cannot* be so recognized is undetermined, as is the question of whether fetal serum would allow prenatal diagnosis.

Table 21.2. Immunological deficiency disorders

Hypogammaglobulinaemia, Bruton type	X-linked recessive
Hypogammaglobulinaemia, Swiss type	Autosomal recessive and X-linked recessive
Combined immunodeficiency due to:	
Adenosine deaminase deficiency	Autosomal recessive
Nucleoside phosphorylase deficiency	Autosomal recessive
Pure thymic dysplasia	Autosomal recessive
Thymic and parathyroid aplasia	
(Di George's syndrome)	Autosomal recessive
Ataxia telangiectasia	Autosomal recessive
Wiskott–Aldrich syndrome	X-linked recessive
Chronic granulomatous disease	X-linked recessive (autosomal recessive)
Complement factor deficiencies	
(various types)	Autosomal recessive

The autosomal recessive combined immunodeficiency due to adenosine deaminase deficiency can be recognized prenatally in cultured amniotic cells.

Disorders of the complement system[9] form a sequence of recessively inherited defects, some characterized by immune deficiency, others being symptomless. An exception is the dominantly inherited C'_1 esterase inhibitor deficiency, responsible for *hereditary angioedema*. In view of the potentially lethal laryngeal problems and the success of preventive and acute therapy, it is important for all close relatives of a patient with this disorder to be carefully checked for the deficiency.

Haemophilia

Haemophilia represents a major genetic counselling problem, and this is likely to grow since most haemophilic males now reach adult life with only moderate disability and frequently reproduce. Both major forms of haemophilia are X-linked, *haemophilia A* resulting from a deficiency of Factor VIII, while in *haemophilia B* (Christmas disease) whose locus is not closely linked, the deficiency is of Factor IX. It is now recognized that Factor VIII is a compound molecule, with one part of small molecular weight determined by the X-linked locus defective in haemophilia A, while the large molecular weight portion is controlled by an autosomal locus, defective in the autosomal dominant disorder *Von Willebrand's disease.*

Genetic advice for males affected with haemophilia (A or B) is straightforward, though mistakes are often made. As with any X-linked recessive disorder, all sons will be healthy, as will their descendants; all daughters will be carriers. It is unnecessary and often misleading for such daughters to have tests of carrier detection, since whatever results these give, the daughter of an affected male *must* be a carrier. An affected female can only occur if an affected male marries a carrier (an exceptionally rare event), or if there is a sex chromosome abnormality such as Turner's (XO) syndrome.

Advice for definite carriers is also clear, there being a 50 per cent risk of sons being affected and the same for daughters being carriers (*see* Chapter 2). The main problems in counselling lie in determining how great is the chance of woman at risk being a carrier, and this is of particular importance if decisions are to be made regarding fetal sexing and prenatal diagnosis.

The risk of being a carrier will depend on:

1. The prior genetic risk.
2. Other genetic information.
3. The results of carrier detection studies.

The use of this information is similar to the situation in Duchenne muscular dystrophy (Chapter 9) and the general approach to the subject for X-linked diseases is discussed in Chapter 2 and 5. It cannot be too strongly stressed that to use information provided by Factor VIII assays in isolation is erroneous and misleading — just as it is to use genetic information without taking into account available results of carrier detection. The different types of information must be correctly combined.

Most laboratories concerned with haemophilia A use a combination of two assays — a functional assay of Factor VIII which is variably reduced in carriers, and an immunological assay which is usually normal. The ratio of these results gives the most sensitive guide to carrier detection; about 70 per cent of carriers can be confidently identified, but as with Duchenne dystrophy, results in the normal range are less easy to interpret. The most satisfactory solution is to use a table of odds (as in Duchenne dystrophy) so that any level of laboratory result can be used to give a particular set of odds for or against being a carrier. This is *not* the actual risk to the individual, but can be combined with genetic information to give this value. Unfortunately, many haemophilia centres are reluctant to use the information in this way, preferring to rely on laboratory data, while ignoring genetic risks. An excellent review by Graham[10] should serve as an example to them and to others. Data for haemophilia B are less satisfactory, but the general approach is the same.

Isolated cases of haemophilia are as much a problem as are isolated cases of Duchenne dystrophy. It is not known what proportion represent new mutations, and there have been suggestions that the great majority of mothers of such cases are carriers. Until the situation is clarified it is wise to assume a high prior risk (at least 80 per cent) of the mother of an isolated case being a carrier; this means that only those with extremely favourable carrier testing results will be able to be given a low final risk.

Women who are definite carriers, or where the risk of this has been shown to be high, have the option of fetal sexing of pregnancies, with termination of a male pregnancy. As discussed in Chapter 6 most couples find this unsatisfactory, especially if the risk of the woman being a carrier is only moderate. However, the recent development of an immunoassay for the low molecular weight component of Factor VIII (absent in haemophilia A) has given the possibility for specific prenatal diagnosis of an affected male fetus if a fetal serum sample can be obtained free from contamination with maternal blood[11, 12]. This has proved a major advance in the control of haemophilia, but the high-risk nature of this type of procedure makes it all the more important that carriers are correctly identified beforehand.

Other Coagulation Disorders

Von Willebrand's disease, as previously mentioned, is usually autosomal dominant, though a very rare, severe recessive form also exists. Deficiencies of numerous other coagulation factors have been recognized, including fibrinogen and prothrombin. All are autosomal recessive. A variety of forms of thrombocytopenia have also been recognized, showing various modes of inheritance, but an X-linked recessive form is the best recognized.

References

1. Kan Y. W. and Dozy A. (1978) Antenatal diagnosis of sickle-cell anaemia by DNA analysis of amniotic fluid cells. *Lancet* 2, 910–912.
2. Stamatoyannopoulos G. (1973) Problems of screening and counseling in the haemoglobinopathies. Excerpta Medica International Congress Series No. 297. pp. 14–15.
3. Weatherall D. J. and Clegg J. B. (1972) *The Thalassaemia Syndromes.* Oxford, Blackwell.
4. Huehns E. R. (1979) Antenatal diagnosis in beta thalassaemia. In: Harper P. S. and Muir J. (ed.), *Advanced Medicine* 15, London, Pitman.
5. Jacob H. S., Ruby A., Overland E. S. et al. (1971) Abnormal membrane protein of red blood cells in hereditary spherocytosis. *J. Clin. Invest.* 50, 1800–1805.
6. Clarke C. A. (1975) *Rhesus Haemolytic Disease.* Selected papers and extracts. Lancaster, MTP.
7. Mourant A. E., Kopeć A. C. and Domaniewska-Sobczak (1978) *Blood Groups and Diseases.* London, Oxford University Press.
8. Guttler F., Seakins J. W. T. and Harkness R. A. (ed.), (1979) *Inborn Errors of Immunity and Phagocytosis.* Lancaster, MTP.
9. Kohler P. F. (1978) The human complement system. In: Samter M. (ed.), *Immunological Diseases.* Boston, Little, Brown. pp. 244–280.
10. Graham J. B. (1979) Genotype assignment in the haemophilias. *Clin. Haematol.* 8, 115–145.

11. Peake I. R. and Bloom A. L. (1978) Immunoradiometric assay of procoagulant factor VIII antigen in plasma and serum and its reduction in haemophilia. *Lancet* 1, 473–475.
12. Mibashan R. S., Rodeck C. H., Thumpston J. K. et al. (1979) Plasma assay of fetal factor VIIIC and IX for prenatal diagnosis of haemophilia. *Lancet* 1, 1309–1311.

CHAPTER TWENTY-TWO

Genetic Risks in Cancer

Genetic counselling may be needed in families where cancer has occurred for a variety of reasons. In a few instances there is a clear familial aggregation with potentially high risks to relatives. In a much larger number the risks are low, but there is fear and concern that other family members might be affected. Finally, the development of malignancy may be associated with an underlying syndrome that itself follows a specific pattern of inheritance.

Many of the individual tumours of particular organs have already been mentioned in previous chapters. The main groups that need to be considered are:

1. Tumours following Mendelian inheritance.
2. Genetic syndromes predisposing to malignancy.
3. Embryonal and childhood tumours.
4. Common malignant tumours of later life.

A clear general review of the genetic aspects of cancer has been provided by Schimke (1978).

Table 22.1. Tumours following Mendelian inheritance

Type	Inheritance	Comments
Retinoblastoma	Autosomal dominant	*See* p. 191
Wilms' tumour (nephroblastoma)	Autosomal dominant	*See* below
Neurofibromatosis	Autosomal dominant	*See* p. 249
Bilateral acoustic neuromas	Autosomal dominant	*See* p. 201
Tuberous sclerosis	Autosomal dominant	*See* p. 144
Von Hippel–Lindau syndrome	Autosomal dominant	
Basal cell naevus syndrome	Autosomal dominant	
Malignant melanoma	Autosomal dominant	Occasional families only
Kaposi's sarcoma	Autosomal dominant	Occasional families only
Self-healing keratoacanthoma	Autosomal dominant	
Multiple endocrine adenomatosis	Autosomal dominant	Two types (*see* p. 229)
Adenocarcinomatosis (cancer family syndrome)	Autosomal dominant	Two types (*see* p. 247)
Oesophageal cancer with tylosis	Autosomal dominant	*See* p. 213
Polyposis syndromes	Autosomal dominant	Several types (*see* p. 217
Ovarian dysgerminoma	Autosomal dominant	Occasional families only

Tumours following Mendelian Inheritance

Although individually rare, the number of Mendelian tumours is considerable (*Table* 22.1) and there is little doubt that many cases are missed from lack of careful history taking in what initially may appear to be an ordinary 'garden variety' non-familial neoplasm. It can be seen that almost all these conditions follow autosomal dominant inheritance and so far no chromosomal or biochemical basis has been found for them. Identification and surveillance of relatives at risk should be one of the major objectives of any genetic register system.

'Cancer Families'

This term has been used for rare, but well documented families in which malignant tumours of a variety of types occur within a family and follow an autosomal dominant pattern. There appear to be at least two separate forms of this disorder. In one, 'adenocarcinomatosis', the tumours are most commonly of stomach, colon, pancreas, breast and other glandular organs, together with ovarian cancer[1]. In the second, the commonest tumours are lymphomas, leukaemias, sarcomas, cerebral tumours and breast cancers[2].

Definite examples are extremely rare, but it is likely that a proportion of lesser concentrations of tumours may also represent these syndromes. Unfortunately, no independent diagnostic aid exists to recognize this important group or to identify the family members at risk. A parallel situation is seen in the different forms of multiple endocrine adenomatosis (p. 229).

Table 22.2. Mendelian syndromes predisposing to malignancy

Syndrome	Inheritance	Type of neoplasm
Xeroderma pigmentosum	Autosomal recessive	Various skin tumours
Fanconi's pancytopenia	Autosomal recessive	Leukaemias
Ataxia telangiectasia	Autosomal recessive	Leukaemias and carcinomas
Bloom's syndrome	Autosomal recessive	Leukaemias
Chediak–Higashi syndrome	Autosomal recessive	Lymphomas
Werner's syndrome	Autosomal recessive	Various
Dyskeratosis congenita	X-linked recessive	Pharyngeal and oesophageal cancer
Wiskott–Aldrich syndrome	X-linked recessive	Leukaemias, lymphomas
Sclerotylosis	Autosomal dominant	Epithelial and adenocarcinomas

Genetic Syndromes predisposing to Malignancy

In contrast to the dominantly inherited specific tumours, the majority of Mendelian syndromes showing a generalized tendency to malignancy follow autosomal recessive inheritance. Some of these have already been shown to be inborn errors of DNA repair and it is likely that others will prove to have a comparable basis.

It is likely that at least some of the syndromes in this group will prove amenable to prenatal diagnosis when more specific biochemical tests are available. This is already feasible for xeroderma pigmentosum.

A potentially important observation is that heterozygotes for these rare recessive disorders may be at increased risk of developing malignancy. There appears to be a three to six-fold increase of overall malignancies in heterozygotes for ataxia telangiectasia and possibly an increase in Fanconi's pancytopenia heterozygotes[3]. The relevance of this extends beyond the families of affected homozygotes since the great majority of heterozygotes for these genes will never produce an affected homozygote and are most unlikely to be recognized.

Embryonal and Childhood Cancer
When known genetic syndromes are excluded, the overall risk of malignancy in childhood is around 1 in 600. A recent study[4] has examined the risk of malignancy occurring in sibs and has shown that it is doubled (1 in 300), with most cases concordant for the same neoplasm. The relative increases in risk divided into the major groups of leukaemias, lymphomas and other malignancies are given below:

		Proband		
		Leukaemia	Lymphoma	Other malignancy
	Leukaemia	X 2·3	X 2·3	X 1·3
Sib	Lymphoma	X 2·9	X 5·4	X 0·7
	Other malignancy	X 1·2	X 0·6	X 2·7
	Total	X 1·7	X 1·7	X 2·0

It would seem reasonable to use this estimate for the various rare forms of childhood cancer where individual data are not yet available, where no other cases of childhood cancer have occurred, and where a clear genetic basis for the neoplasm is not known to exist. Sarcomas, neuroblastoma and cerebral tumours of childhood all fall in this category.

Wilms Tumour (Nephroblastoma)
Incidence is 1 in 20 000. Survival into adult life has only recently become usual, but it is now clear that the situation is comparable to that seen in *retinoblastoma* (*see* p. 191) and that an appreciable proportion of cases follows Mendelian inheritance including almost all those with bilateral tumours. Unfortunately, it is often impossible to separate this group from the other cases, and as with retinoblastoma penetrance is incomplete (around 60 per cent). Schimke has estimated the following risks for

relatives of patients with Wilms tumour, based on the data of Knudson and Strong[5]:

Affected member	Risk for subsequent children
Parent with bilateral tumours	
Parent with unilateral tumour + affected relative	30%
Parent unaffected; 2 affected children	
Parent with unilateral tumour	10%
Sib with bilateral tumours	10%
Sib with unilateral tumour	5%

In addition, Wilms tumour may be associated with aniridia (recurrence risks as above) and may occur in several dominantly inherited syndromes with hemi-hypertrophy, the Beckwith—Wiedemann syndrome and with other embryonal tumours in one form of the 'cancer family syndrome'. Further problems, also similar to retinoblastoma, are a probable raised risk of tumours elsewhere in later life, not entirely explicable by radiation treatment.

Neuroblastoma
In contrast to Wilms tumour, the great majority of cases are sporadic, but poorer survival means that adequate data are not available for the offspring of affected patients. In the few two-generation families known, the parent has usually had spontaneous maturation of the tumour. The risk for further sibs of an isolated case is unlikely to exceed 1 per cent and is probably nearer the 1 in 300 risk found overall for sibs in childhood cancer. Where two sibs, or parent and child are affected, the risk for further sibs is much greater, probably that of an incompletely penetrant dominant gene, about 30 per cent as for Wilms tumour.

Leukaemias
The great majority of cases of all types of leukaemia do not seem to have a hereditary basis.

Acute leukaemia is most commonly seen in childhood, where it accounts for a major proportion of all malignancies. The risks for sibs have been given above and amount only to a doubling of risk for leukaemia with a 1 in 300 chance of childhood malignancy overall. The various chromosomal abnormalities described in blood cells[6], appear to be a consequence of the disorder, rather than representing a primary genetic abnormality. Rare clusters of acute leukaemia may represent an environmental factor; however, leukaemia may be a complication of a number of primary genetic disorders including immune deficiencies, DNA repair defects and Down's syndrome. No data are yet available for the offspring of the increasing number of survivors. Risks of leukaemia are likely to be small, but an increase in other abnormalities as a result of therapy cannot be excluded.

Chronic myeloid leukaemia carries little risk to relatives; although the 'Philadelphia' chromosome abnormality − a partial deletion of chromosome 22 resulting from translocation of part of it onto chromosome 9 − is a constant finding in most cases, this is a somatic event, not affecting the germ line.

Chronic lymphatic leukaemia likewise rarely recurs in a family, but a small number of multi-generation families makes it possible that a dominantly inherited form exists among the much commoner non-genetic cases.

Lymphomas

As with leukaemias, most cases are sporadic; clustering is suggestive of an infective agent and may well not be genetic. The same primary genetic diseases as predispose to leukaemias (except for Down's syndrome) may also be responsible for lymphomas, and the same reservations about the offspring of 'cured' patients apply. Study of the sibs of childhood cases shows a five-fold increase in risk for lymphomas, but the overall risk of childhood malignancy is still only around 1 in 300.

Histiocytosis

This confused and heterogeneous group contains several Mendelian disorders presenting in childhood − adult cases appear to be non-genetic.

1. Letterer−Siwe disease. Autosomal recessive. Rapidly progressive and fatal.

2. X-linked histiocytosis. X-linked recessive. Clinically variable and may be accompanied by immune deficiency.

Common Cancers of Later Life

While the great majority of these are not familial, individual families showing concentrations of particular tumours have frequently been reported, and present a difficult counselling problem. Rare Mendelian syndromes (e.g. polyposis coli) must be carefully excluded, as must conditions giving different tumour types, such as the 'cancer family syndrome' (adenocarcinomatosis). Environmental agents may give familial clustering, which may be maternally transmitted, e.g. hepatitis B in hepatoma. Most commonly none of these factors can be identified, and it is impossible to be certain whether the family concentration is the result of chance, of a concentration of polygenic factors, or the action of a major gene.

Where specific studies have been done, the risk to first-degree relatives has usually been found to be increased about threefold where only one family member is affected. This has been shown for gastric and colonic cancer, and for bronchial carcinoma. It is relevant that in this last case, genetic and environmental factors interact in a more than additive fashion.

Thus in a carefully controlled study, heavy smokers with an affected first-degree relative had a fourteen-fold increase in risk, whereas each factor alone only increased the risk threefold[7]. Studies of aryl carbon hydroxylase may help to predict high-risk individuals[8].

The following situations are likely to increase the risk significantly:

1. Two sibs affected, or parent + sib. In the absence of other information, and using the basis of polygenic determination with low penetrance, an increase around eightfold seems probable.

2. More family members than the above affected. Here it becomes so difficult to distinguish the situation from autosomal dominant inheritance, that a risk approaching 50 per cent for offspring of an affected person or sib of multiple affected sibs seems reasonable. Unlike the firmly established autosomal dominant situation, however, one cannot exclude risk to the offspring of unaffected family members. Unfortunately, no empiric data exist for this, and the theoretical basis is too uncertain to warrant more than a rough estimate.

3. Multiple primary tumours. This has been found to increase the risk to relatives in the case of colonic cancer, and may well do so for other tumours.

4. Risk to twins. Concordance for both monozygotic and dizygotic twins is low for most common cancers.

Where no data are available (as in the case of most tumours) it seems reasonable to use the theoretical risks predicted for polygenic inheritance as given in *Table* 3.3, p. 52. The 'low heritability' category is probably the most appropriate.

References
1. Lynch H. and Krush A. J. (1973) Differential diagnosis of the cancer family syndrome. *Surg. Gynecol. Obstet.* **136**, 221–224.
2. Li F. P. and Fraumeni J. F. (1975) Familial breast cancer, soft tissue sarcomas and other neoplasms. *Ann. Int. Med.* **83**, 833–834.
3. Swift M. (1976) Malignant disease in heterozygous carriers. *Birth Defects* **12**, 133–144.
4. Draper G. J., Heaf M. M. and Wilson L. M. K. (1977) Occurrence of childhood cancers among sibs and estimation of familial risks. *J. Med. Genet.* **14**, 81–90.
5. Knudson A. G. and Strong L. C. (1972) Mutation and cancer: a model for Wilms' tumour of the kidney. *J. Natl Cancer Inst.* **48**, 313–324.
6. Rowley D. (1976) The role of cytogenetics in haematology. *Blood* **48**, 1–7.
7. Tokuhata G. K. and Lilienfeld A. M. (1963) Familial aggregation of lung cancer in humans. *J. Natl. Cancer Inst.* **30**, 289–312.
8. Emery A. E. H., Anand R., Denford N. et al. (1978) Aryl-hydrocarbon-hydroxylase inducibility in patients with cancer. *Lancet* **1**, 470–471.

Further Reading
Harper P. S. (1973) Heredity and gastrointestinal tumours. *Clin. Gastroenterol.* **2**, 675–701.
Mulvihill J. J., Miller R. W. and Fraumeni J. F. (ed.), (1977) *Genetics of Human Cancer. Progress in Cancer Research and Therapy.* New York, Raven Press.
Schimke R. N. (1978) *Genetics and Cancer in Man.* Edinburgh, Churchill Livingstone.

CHAPTER TWENTY-THREE

Environmental Hazards

At first sight this subject might seem to bear little relation to genetic counselling, but in practice there are several reasons why environmental agents and their risks need consideration. First, they may come into the differential diagnosis of malformation syndromes, e.g. congenital rubella must be considered among the possible causes of congenital cataract, and the recurrence risks will be greatly affected if such an agent can be confirmed or firmly excluded. Secondly, many agents causing fetal damage in pregnancy may also cause harmful mutations — radiation is the prime example. Thirdly, enquiry may be made as to whether cytogenetic or prenatal diagnostic tests may be of help in confirming or excluding fetal damage.

Three groups of agents will briefly be discussed here:
1. Congenital infections.
2. Drugs believed to be teratogenic.
3. Radiation and other potential mutagenic agents.

Table 23.1. Congenital infections

Agent	Common defects
Rubella	Cataract, deafness, congenital heart disease
Cytomegalovirus	Microcephaly, chorioretinitis, hepatosplenomegaly
Hepatitis virus	Biliary atresia (?), hepatic damage
Other viruses	*See text*
Toxoplasma	Chorioretinitis, microcephaly, hepatosplenomegaly
Syphilis	Facial and other bony abnormalities, keratitis

Congenital Infections

Table 23.1 lists the major types. Among these *congenital syphilis* is rarely seen now in Western populations; overwhelmingly the most important is *congenital rubella*[1]. It is to be hoped that systematic immunization will soon make this also a rarity.

The principal malformations seen in congenital rubella include cataracts, nerve deafness, congenital heart defects (commonly patent ductus arteriosus) and microcephaly with mental retardation. Since congenital rubella may occur in the absence of overt maternal infection, it is a condition that must be considered seriously in the differential diagnosis of any syndrome where these abnormalities occur.

The risk to a subsequent pregnancy after a child with congenital rubella has been born is negligible; the critical information usually required is the risk to a current pregnancy in which the mother has developed or has been exposed to the infection. Where the mother is already known to have immunity, on the basis of immunization or previous serological tests, the risk to the fetus is exceedingly low. Where this information is not available it is extremely difficult to obtain rapid direct evidence for fetal infection or lack of it, though it is likely that suitable tests may soon become available on amniotic fluid; at present negative cultures and immune titres on amniotic fluid are not adequate to exclude infection.

The only reliable information that can currently be used to predict risks is that infection in the first month of pregnancy carries an extremely high risk of abnormality (around 60 per cent), which falls to about 25 per cent for infection in the second month and about 8 per cent in the third month. Risks are small for abnormality after infection in the second trimester, and negligible after this. Indications for termination of pregnancy are clearly strong in the early stages, but the decision may be difficult around the third month, or if dates are uncertain. More specific tests will be of great help. Careful examination of an apparently normal infant at risk (especially audiometry) is important to exclude minor degrees of damage.

Cytomegalovirus Infection [2]

Microcephaly with mental retardation, chorioretinitis, deafness, hepatosplenomegaly and purpuric rash are common features. Maternal infection is often asymptomatic and no preventive measures, apart from evidence of known or potential sources of infection, are available.

Other Viral Infections [3]

Although there have been many suggested associations, evidence for the teratogenicity of other viruses is much less well established than the above. It is possible that *hepatitis virus* may be involved in at least some cases of biliary atresia. Maternal transmission of this virus may produce familial chronic liver disease in later life in susceptible individuals. *Herpes simplex* virus may be associated with some cases of microcephaly, while influenza virus has been claimed to be responsible for some of the cyclical peaks of malformations such as neural tube defects. Live viral vaccines, while obviously undesirable in pregnancy, have in fact only occasionally produced any evidence of fetal damage.

Toxoplasmosis [4]

Chorioretinitis, CNS involvement with convulsions, hepatosplenomegaly and rash are the main features. Maternal infection is often asymptomatic and is usually from domestic animals, in particular cats.

Drugs and Malformations

Since the epidemic of limb defects due to thalidomide[5] there has not only been stringent testing of new agents for teratogenicity, but many studies have investigated possible associations. In fact the number of *specific* malformation syndromes clearly related to individual drugs is extremely small (*Table* 23.2); much more difficult to assess are situations

Table 23.2. Drugs with teratogenic effect

Definite
Thalidomide
Warfarin
Alcohol
Aminopterin and methotrexate
Probable
Phenytoin
Trimethadione
Lithium
Possible
Sex hormones
Ergotamine
Anaesthetic gases
Industrial chemicals

where a commonly used drug (e.g. an anticonvulsant) appears to be associated with an increased incidence of certain malformations, and where the type of malformation is either variable or commonly seen in the absence of the agent. It is likely that most of the associations still to be discovered are in this latter group, where proof of a causal relationship is exceedingly difficult to obtain.

Despite the small number of firm teratogenic syndromes due to drugs, it is clearly prudent for all drugs that are not strictly essential to be avoided in pregnancy, and indeed avoided by all women who are at risk of conceiving. Avoidance of cigarette smoking and the taking of a nutritious balanced diet are additional commonsense factors that are desirable even in the absence of specific evidence. General advice of this type can often be given in conjunction with genetic counselling since most couples known to be at increased risk for abnormality in the offspring will be anxious to do anything possible to reduce this risk.

Thalidomide [5]

A generation of children with thalidomide-induced limb defects and other abnormalities is now growing up, particularly in continental Europe, but also in Great Britain. Where the relationship with thalidomide is clear cut there should, of course, be no increased risk of abnormalities in the offspring of these patients, but it seems likely that some dominantly inherited limb reduction defects may have mistakenly been attributed to thalidomide, in which case affected children may well be born. The recessively inherited pseudothalidomide or Roberts' syndrome may also be confused.

Warfarin [6]

This has been clearly associated with a syndrome identical to the severe form of chondrodysplasia punctata (Conradi's disease). Although occurring only in a small proportion of exposed pregnancies, there is a high fetal and perinatal loss overall, so it seems quite clear that warfarin and related anticoagulants are undesirable in women who are pregnant or at risk of becoming so. In one case known to the author the pregnancy resulted from stopping oral contraceptives which had resulted in a venous thrombosis, warfarin then being used for therapy — a double iatrogenic misfortune.

Alcohol [7]

There seems no doubt as to the existence of a syndrome of abnormal facies, reduced somatic and brain growth, mental retardation and congenital heart disease in mothers with a high alcohol intake in pregnancy. There is, however, real doubt as to how common the disorder is and whether lesser degrees of alcohol consumption are teratogenic. In Britain, in contrast to America and Sweden, the syndrome seems to be exceedingly uncommon despite awareness of its existence; the difference seems to be a genuine one.

Phenytoin [8]

A moderately specific syndrome of low birth weight, mental retardation, unusual facies with hypertelorism, congenital heart defects and hypoplastic digits appears to occur rarely. An overall increase in the incidence of cleft lip and palate has also been suggested [9], but is not so clearly attributable to this drug in particular.

Trimethadione [10]

Again there appears to be an occasional specific combination of congenital heart defects, genito-urinary abnormalities, unusual facies with synophrys, and mental retardation, with a considerable increase (possibly as high as 20 per cent) in congenital heart disease in isolation.

Lithium

Lithium, an increasingly used agent in affective disorders, has now been convincingly associated with the occurrence of congenital disease, in particular Ebstein's anomaly [11].

Sex Hormones

The use of female sex hormones in early pregnancy for prevention of threatened abortion and for treatment of infertility has declined, partly due to concern regarding fetal abnormalities. A general increase in common malformations has been suspected, but in particular the 'VATER' group of anomalies (see p. 164) seems to be specifically related in many cases to maternal hormone treatment [12]. Doubt still exists as to whether hormone pregnancy tests are in any way teratogenic, and as to whether conception while on oral contraceptives is harmful. An increased malformation rate has been seen following ovulation-inducing drugs, but whether this is a direct effect, or related to the frequently associated twinning or the underlying cause of the infertility, is unknown. Alberman [13] gives a clear review of this confused topic.

Immunosuppresive and Cytotoxic Drugs

Increasing numbers of women are reproducing while on these drugs for previously lethal diseases or following renal transplantation. So far, few obvious abnormalities have been found in pregnancies going to term; aminopterin and its derivative methotrexate have been associated with a specific severe connective tissue syndrome [14]. Problems in this group are perhaps more likely to arise from their mutagenic properties (see below).

Industrial and Other Chemicals

Despite widespread and reasonable concern, actual evidence for human teratogenic effects is scanty. Claims for increased abnormalities after deliberate mass spraying or industrial accidents involving the herbicide 2, 4, 5—T are circumstantial, as is the case for other chemicals such as hair dyes. An effect of inhaled anaesthetic gases by pregnant operating theatre staff and anaesthetists seems more soundly based [15]; an increase in spontaneous abortions and in a variety of common malformations was seen, rather than any particular combination.

Genetic Effects of Radiation [16, 17]

A large amount of work has been done on the population effects of accidental, diagnostic and therapeutic radiation. A clear and simple review is given by Emery [18]. However, we are concerned here with the effects on a particular conception or pregnancy.

Two separate situations must be considered, which are often confused by those requesting information:

1. Mutagenic effects, resulting in damage to germ cells *before* fertilization.

2. Teratogenesis, i.e. damage to the developing embryo.

Mutagenesis must be considered separately for the sexes, since the method of germ cell formation in each is entirely different. In males, animal experiments have shown two major classes of abnormality:

a. Major chromosomal abnormalities, occurring mainly in the offspring conceived a few days or weeks after irradiation.

b. An increased incidence of point mutations, persisting in offspring conceived long after irradiation has been given.

For the human male one can probably draw the following conclusions regarding risks to offspring:

1. Diagnostic irradiation is of little significance.

2. Conception in the few months after therapeutic irradiation (especially of the gonads) is unwise; amniocentesis is advisable should pregnancy occur in order to detect chromosomal defects. The same probably applies when a man is or has recently been taking cytotoxic drugs or other known chemical mutagens.

3. A variable period of infertility is common after gonadal irradiation (and with cytotoxic drugs), but should not be relied upon.

4. Long-term risks for a pregnancy conceived many months or years after irradiation are small, and result mainly from increased dominant mutations, which are unlikely to be detected by amniocentesis. However, the incidence of such abnormalities is low (not over 1 per cent).

In women the oocyte is especially radiation sensitive around the time of fertilization; outside this period risks are likely to be similar to or less than for males. Diagnostic radiation is unlikely to be a significant risk factor for future children of an individual woman, though unnecessary exposure clearly should be avoided to avoid even a small population increase in point mutations and chromosome defects.

Irradiation during pregnancy is a somewhat different problem, and is the commonest cause of referral for genetic counselling. Such irradiation is almost always diagnostic, with a dose of 1 rad or less; it is usually inadvertant and given in the earliest weeks of pregnancy before a pregnancy has been recognized. It is not uncommon for such irradiation to be given during the course of investigation for infertility, and the combination of a wanted pregnancy with the feelings of guilt shared by patient and doctor that radiation exposure should have occurred may produce considerable anxiety.

Until recently termination of pregnancy has been frequently advised in such a situation, but it is likely that the risks to the fetus have been considerably overestimated and are in fact very small for diagnostic levels of radiation. A valuable review by Mole[19] concludes that after 1 rad (the upper limit for most diagnostic radiation) the total added risk to the fetus is unlikely to exceed 1 in 1000, this risk being partly for malformations, partly for mental retardation and childhood cancer. In such circumstances neither termination nor amniocentesis seem warranted, though it is probably wise to stress the relatively frequent occurrence of abnormalities in the general population, since there is a real danger that any such occurrence will be attributed to the radiation.

Information on the risks of heavy doses of radiation has come mainly from follow-up of Japanese atomic bomb casualties[16]. At levels over 50 rad there is a clear and dose related increase in mental retardation in such exposed pregnancies (10 per cent at 200 rad). Since amniocentesis or other prenatal procedures are unlikely to exclude this, there is a strong indication for termination of pregnancy. Such an exposure is rare in a peacetime situation and would probably be associated with severe maternal illness anyway.

References

1. Dudgeon J. A. (1967) Maternal rubella and its effect on the foetus. *Arch. Dis. Child.* 42, 110−125.
2. Dudgeon J. A. (1971) Cytomegalovirus infection. *Arch. Dis. Child.* 46, 581−583.
3. Hurley R. (1978) Antenatal infections associated with fetal malformations. In: Scrimgeour J. B. (ed.), *Towards the Prevention of Fetal Malformation.* Edinburgh University Press, pp. 101−119.
4. Desmonts G. and Couvreur J. (1974) Congenital toxoplasmosis. A prospective study of 378 pregnancies. *N. Engl. J. Med.* 290, 1110−1116.
5. Lenz W. and Knapp K. (1962) Thalidomide embryopathy. *Arch. Environ. Health* 5, 100−105.
6. Holzgreve W., Carey J. C. and Hall B. D. (1976) Warfarin induced fetal abnormalities. *Lancet* 2, 914.
7. Jones K. L. and Smith D. W. (1975) The fetal alcohol syndrome. *Teratology* 12, 1−10.
8. Hanson J. W. and Smith D. W. (1975) The fetal hydantoin syndrome. *J. Pediat.* 87, 285−290.
9. Meadow W. R. (1970) Congenital abnormalities and anticonvulsant drugs. *Proc. R. Soc. Med.* 63, 12−13.
10. Zackai E., Mellmann M. and Neiderer B. (1975) The fetal trimethadione syndrome. *J. Pediat.* 87, 280−284.
11. Nora J. J., Nora A. H. and Toews W. H. (1974) Lithium, Ebstein's anomaly and other congenital heart defects. *Lancet* 2, 594−595.
12. Nora J. J. and Nora A. H. (1978) *Genetics and Counseling in Cardiovascular Diseases.* Springfield, Thomas, pp. 142−144.
13. Alberman E. (1978) Fertility drugs and contraceptive agents. In: Scrimgeour J. B. (ed.), *Towards the Prevention of Fetal Malformation.* Edinburgh University Press, pp. 89−100.
14. Milunsky A., Graef J. W. and Gaynor M. F. (1968) Methotrexate-induced congenital malformations. *J. Pediat.* 72, 790−795.
15. Cohen E. N., Brown B. W., Bruce D. L. et al. (1974) Occupational disease among operating room personnel. *Anesthesiology* 41, 321−340.
16. UNSCEAR Report (1972) Ionizing radiation: levels and effects, Vol. 11, Anex E. New York, United Nations.
17. Proceedings of the Symposium on the Effects of Low Radiation Doses on the Maturation of the Developing (Human) Ovum and Foetus (1968) *Br. J. Radiol.* 41, 714−722.

18. Emery A. E. H. (ed.) (1979) Radiation and human heredity. In: *Elements of Medical Genetics*. Edinburgh, Churchill-Livingstone.
19. Mole R. H. (1979) Radiation effects on prenatal development and their radiological significance. *Br. J. Radiol.* **52**, 89–101.

Further Reading
Congenital Malformations, Notes and Comments (1971) Chicago, Year Book.
Wilson J. G. and Clarke Frazer F. (ed.) (1977) *Handbook of Teratology* (Vols. 1–4). New York, Plenum.

III. Conclusion

CHAPTER TWENTY-FOUR

Genetic Counselling and Society

The primary aim of this book has been to provide information that will help particular families in which a genetic disorder exists or is at risk of occurring. Throughout the book the family, at times nuclear, at others extended, has been the unit under consideration, and it is hoped that both the general discussions and the more specific information in the later chapters will have helped the reader answer most of the problems that confront him as well as alerting him to some of the pitfalls and unsolved problems that exist.

Most doctors will, however, not be fully satisfied by dealing with these individual problems in isolation, but will wish to place them in the more general context of prevention and to know how far they can extend these individual instances of genetic counselling towards the wider prevention of inherited disorders in the population that they serve. Thus a general practitioner may wonder how his genetic counselling is contributing to reducing the general burden of genetic disease in his practice population, while a neurologist might ask the same question about specific disorders that he commonly encounters, such as Duchenne dystrophy or Huntington's chorea. The medical geneticist in particular, will be anxious to learn whether the genetic counselling which is his major day-to-day occupation is having any effect on the patterns of genetic disease in the population, as well as on the individual families that he sees.

These wider population aspects have so far received very little emphasis in this book, in part because the author's view is that the primary duty of a physician is to individuals and their immediate families, in part because the general aspects can only be approached through study of the particular. However, it would be entirely wrong to suggest, as is sometimes done, that these wider aspects are not the concern of those undertaking genetic counselling; to take such a view would be as short-sighted as it would have been for the 19th century physician to insist that only the individual case of typhoid fever was his concern, not the broader epidemiology of the disease.

Even if the reader is not curious about the wider effects of genetic counselling, these are likely to be forced upon his notice; a couple where the husband is haemophilic may press for termination of a healthy, but carrier female pregnancy on grounds of 'not wishing to hand on the gene to future generations'. Critics of a screening programme for phenylketonuria may argue that treating such patients may cause an increase in the disease in future. Administrators may wish to know the projected future incidence of spina bifida or Duchenne dystrophy in the light of screening or counselling programmes. Such questions all necessitate an accurate knowledge of the effects of counselling for a particular disorder on the population as a whole. The following paragraphs discuss some of the points that must be taken into consideration.

Whom does Genetic Counselling Reach?

Anyone regularly involved in genetic counselling will be under no illusions that his advice is reaching all the individuals who need it. In general, he will be seeing a small segment of the community which is both sufficiently motivated and sufficiently articulate to ask for referral or to ask the type of question to make their own doctor either answer them or arrange for referral. Inevitably, this means that the less privileged, generally with the greatest need, are less well served. Even in a system like the British National Health Service, where finance is no barrier, the same situation applies, and at present it seems likely that genetic counselling is only dealing with the 'tip of the iceberg', even in those situations where it could have a much more profound effect.

Improved awareness of genetic problems among medical and para-medical staff will undoubtedly help, and is the principal aim of this book. This alone, however, is unlikely to have more than a minor effect unless there is a comparable change in the awareness and motivation of the population as a whole. Genetic counselling given to those who do not wish it or who are unaware of the underlying problem is often an unrewarding procedure for physician and patient alike.

The author's view is that genetic counselling will only have its full impact when an awareness of its importance and availability is built into the general education of young people around the school-leaving age. At a time when small families are the rule, it seems essential for those having children to take every possible measure to ensure that those they have will be healthy, and to do so beforehand. At present, public awareness of the subject, largely the result of television, is focused on problems and diagnostic techniques *during* pregnancy – quite the worst time for a rational appreciation of the situation. As a result, there is a real danger at present of increasing the general level of anxiety without any corresponding increase in the overall level of peoples' knowledge.

The next decade should hopefully see a shift of emphasis to the pre-conceptual phase, with genetic counselling forming part of overall health education prior to reproduction. Should this occur, it will markedly increase the demand for counselling on primary clinicians as well as on the specialist genetic counselling services, a further reason why the author feels strongly that all interested clinicians should be involved in the process and that it should not be 'hived off' as an isolated activity.

What Proportion of Genetic Disease is Potentially Preventable?

Even with the most complete ascertainment and cooperation from the population, the prevention of inherited disorders has to rest on the bare facts of the genetic situation. Thus, in such dominantly inherited disorders as Huntington's chorea, where the proportion of new mutations is low, the prospect for prevention is ultimately good, whereas in Apert's syndrome, where almost all cases are new mutations, or even in achondroplasia, where mutations account for 80 per cent of cases, genetic counselling will make little impact on the population incidence of the disorder, since most cases will arise 'out of the blue' into a family that is not known to be at risk.

The same will apply to most autosomal recessive disorders, since the overwhelming majority of the abnormal genes are in healthy heterozygotes, who will not be aware of this unless they marry someone carrying the same harmful gene and have an affected child. Only the small number of second or subsequent cases in a sibship are likely to be preventable unless population screening of heterozygotes is feasible. Such a course is only a practical proposition for the commonest disorders in a population, and where it has been attempted (e.g. haemoglobinopathies, thalassaemias, Tay—Sachs disease) there have been problems of education and acceptance in the population that were much greater than anticipated even in a successful programme, such as that for Tay—Sachs disease in American Jewish communities; in others (e.g. sickle-cell disease) the problems have so far been overwhelming.

X-linked disorders seem at first sight to be a suitable area for prevention in the population, and certainly the testing of the extended family for carrier status is probably one of the most valuable parts of genetic counselling. Even here, however, mutation may form a considerable baseline and efforts at prevention have to be seen in perspective. It is salutary to note than an apparent dramatic decline in new cases of Duchenne dystrophy following systematic carrier studies in Western Australia proved on closer inspection to have reduced the new mutations as much as the familial cases! Further study over a longer period has shown that while familial cases have indeed been reduced, the new mutations are still as common as before[1].

The most valuable group of disorders to be influenced in population terms by genetic counselling are the late onset autosomal dominant disorders in which fertility is little reduced. Huntington's chorea is a notable example, but polycystic kidney disease, myotonic dystrophy and polyposis coli are others. Here the proportion of cases represented by mutation is low (1—2 per cent in Huntington's chorea), so that, *in theory*, the frequency of the disease could be reduced dramatically within a generation if those at high risk of developing the disorder refrained from reproducing.

In practice, this optimistic situation is far from being realized — Huntington's chorea has remained as common as it was when Huntington described it over a century ago, and in the author's population of South Wales, it has shown a relative increase in the present century [2]. In assessing this dismal situation it is easy to be sceptical and say that it is in the nature of people to take no notice and that it is best to leave well alone! In fact, the lack of any decrease in Huntington's chorea reflects the fact that no one has taken the time or trouble to seek out those needing advice, to give support as well as information, and to continue this process over a number of years. The author's own work[3] has shown that if these simple but basic (and arduous) tasks are done, a striking decrease can result (*Fig.* 24.1), which

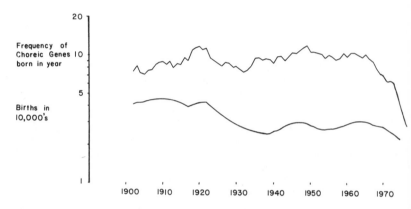

Fig. 24.1. Frequency of choreic genes weighted according to risk compared with births in the related population of Glamorgan and Gwent, 1900–1978, expressed on a log scale. (Five year moving averages used to smooth curves.)

seems likely to be at least in part the consequence of the preventive measures. It should be further noted that this has been possible in the absence of any predictive or prenatal tests, and without 'directive' counselling of those at risk. There seems no reason why other late onset dominant disorders should not respond similarly, and this will become increasingly important as improved treatment of other dominant disorders increases their reproductive potential.

Where the commoner 'polygenic' disorders, and such chromosomal disorders as Down's syndrome are concerned, genetic counselling is less valuable in overall prevention in populations than are screening programmes for those at high risk (e.g. elderly mothers for Down's) or for the whole population (e.g. raised serum alphafetoprotein for neural tube defects). Where genetic counselling is important is in conjunction with such screening programmes, to ensure that those subjected to tests are fully informed, and to put the risks into perspective.

Will Genetic Counselling Increase the Load of Deleterious Genes?

The pessimist is likely to be as wrong as the optimist who hopes to 'wipe out genetic disease' if he tries to generalize indiscriminately. We have already seen that genetic counselling may result in a marked reduction in frequency of both the disease and the gene in certain dominantly inherited disorders, but that in other situations there is little effect. Influences increasing gene frequency are likely to be equally diverse.

Successful treatment of previously fatal or disabling dominant disorders certainly might allow a rapid rise in frequency if accompanied by unrestrained reproduction, though it would be the treatment, rather than genetic counselling that would tend to produce this. Lack of any obvious example where this has happened probably indicates the total lack of medical progress in treating this group of disorders; the only effect of 'advances' has been to make such diseases as the porphyrias more serious by exposing the patients to the hazards of drugs! If treatment of a disorder really proves successful then the problem has probably disappeared anyway.

X-linked disorders where fetal sexing is employed in prenatal diagnosis probably provide the major example where genetic measures might increase the population frequency. By allowing female carriers to have daughters (half of whom will themselves carry the gene) without the risk of having an affected son, it is likely that a steady (though at present undefined) increase will be seen. Direct prenatal diagnosis of affected males would reduce this trend since by avoiding abortion of healthy male fetuses, fewer pregnancies would be needed to reach the desired family size.

A more important potential source of increase in deleterious genes might be expected to arise with the numerous polygenic malformations which in the past were generally fatal but where treatment (usually surgical) now allows a near normal lifespan and fertility. Congenital heart disease, pyloric stenosis, Hirschsprung's disease and hydrocephalus are but a few examples. Although the risks for offspring of such individuals are relatively low (usually under 5 per cent) there is no doubt that in the absence of tests of prenatal detection, reproduction of such individuals will produce a slow, but appreciable rise in the overall level of genetic liability in the population.

Marriage Between Affected Individuals

This is commonly seen in some groups of disorders, such as congenital deafness and blindness, and dwarfism; it may well be increasing as a result of the activity of 'disease specific' lay societies. The genetic risks for couples in particular situations have already been discussed, but worry is sometimes expressed as to the overall effects of such assortative matings on the population level of the particular harmful genes.

In fact, such effects are negligible in the case of rare Mendelian disorders and usually also for the commoner polygenic disorders (e.g. diabetes). The general effect is a redistribution of affected children so that more are likely to be born to affected parents and fewer to unaffected. Thus, although genetic counselling is of great importance for these high-risk couples, their reproduction will have little overall effect on the population frequency of the disease or the gene.

Inbreeding and Outbreeding

Many inbred populations are characterized by high levels of autosomal recessive disorders, and where this is the case, there is no doubt that outbreeding would greatly reduce the frequency of the disease. Thus, a marked increase in the proportion of marriages between Ashkenazi Jews and Gentiles would sharply decrease the incidence of Tay–Sachs disease, especially common in the former. The *gene frequency* would not be decreased, but a greater proportion of the genes would be present in healthy heterozygotes.

Conversely, fragmentation and isolation combined with inbreeding are likely to increase the incidence of autosomal recessive disorders, even when the parent population does not have a particularly high frequency of deleterious genes. Again, it is not the gene frequency but the frequency of affected homozytoes that is increased. Prolonged inbreeding over many generations may actually 'breed out' harmful recessive genes by progressively eliminating them as homozygotes. However, this is not a helpful course to recommend prospectively. The precise effects on gene and phenotype frequencies are thoroughly analysed in a number of books on population genetics; the moral for the clinician should be to beware of generalizations, and to realize that in the great majority of situations the advice given to individual couples may have a profound effect on them and their offspring, but will rarely alter the population structure to a significant extent.

Common Diseases and Traits

Much of the misplaced enthusiasm of the early eugenists was directed towards the reduction of disorders and characteristics considered undesirable such as 'criminality', whose genetic component was often greatly overestimated. Even where the genetic basis was considerable, repressive legislation against reproduction of groups such as epileptics and those of reduced intelligence rightly caused a reaction, so that such laws have almost all been abolished. Most people would agree that it is no part of medical genetic counselling to attempt to alter the overall level in the population of a characteristic such as intelligence, even though its determination may well be largely genetic and it is arguably the most important of all human characteristics. As with most normally distributed characteristics the overall population level is determined predominantly by the actions of the great majority of 'normal' individuals in the middle of the curve. What happens as a result of reproduction at the extremes (both high and low) will be of little overall importance to the genetic structure of the population, even though the consequences to the individual couples may be considerable.

Thus, reproduction of two individuals with non-specific moderate mental retardation is of major importance in terms of risks to the off-spring, but not in terms of the population structure as a whole, and genetic counselling in such a situation is essentially concerned with the first aspect. In the same way 'positive eugenic' efforts by couples of high intelligence to raise the general level of intelligence by having large families are likely to have little overall *genetic* effect, though the social effect of a small number of highly intelligent individuals is undeniably out of all pro-portion to their genetic effect. Only a widespread and continued increase in the family size of the upper ranges of intelligence would be likely to produce a significant genetic change in the population.

In conclusion, when genetic counselling is dealing with the individual family it is often capable of being precise, helpful and profoundly affecting the decisions of individual couples. This is rarely true at the population level and here the clinician should be sceptical that his advice is having any significant effect, either beneficial or adverse, save in a few specific situ-ations. This is perhaps fortunate, for it means that there is rarely any ethical conflict for either physician or patient between the course that is most beneficial for an individual or a family, and that of society as a whole.

Finally, it should be borne in mind that variation is the basis of life and of man's evolution, and that genetic characteristics today considered harmful may not always remain so. The 'thrifty genotype' of the diabetic may once have been associated with advantageous factors and may yet be again in a world with shrinking food resources. The phenylketonuric genotype, recently genetically lethal, is now almost of neutral effect, at least for males, and the advent of successful treatment will undoubtedly ameliorate many other genetic diseases.

Genetic counselling has to be seen as only one part, albeit an important one, of the overall management of the patient and family with a genetic disorder; as was emphasized in the opening paragraphs of this book, it should be an integral part of the work of all interested and informed clinicians, not solely the preserve of a group of specialists. If this book has succeeded in making an appreciable number of clinicians aware of the importance, scope, limitations and pitfalls of genetic counselling in their own work, then it will have amply served its purpose.

References
1. Kakulas B. A. and Hurst P. V. (1977) The muscular dystrophies: results of carrier detection and genetic counselling in Western Australia. *Records of the Adelaide Children's Hospital* 1, 232–243.
2. Harper P. S., Walker D. A., Tyler A. et al. (1979) Huntington's chorea. The basis for long term prevention. *Lancet* 2, 346–349.
3. Harper P. S., Newcombe R., Davies K. et al. Unpublished data.

Appendix

Useful Information in Connection with Genetic Counselling

Various practical items which it is hoped will be of use are listed below. Since this type of information is particularly likely to change, any amended or supplementary details will be welcomed for inclusion in future editions of this book.

Adoption

Specialist agencies that may be helpful in case of difficulty, both for the potential adoptive parent and for the child for adoption with a handicap:

Adoption Resource Exchange (UK),
40 Brunswick Square, London WC1 1AZ.
Parent to Parent Information on Adoption Society (PPIAS) UK,
26 Belsize Grove, London NW3.

Little People of America (USA) and Association for Research into restricted growth (UK) both offer information and help for people with dwarfing conditions wishing to adopt a child with a similar problem.

Genetic Advisory Centres

Almost all regions of the UK now have specialist genetic advisory centres, usually working in close association with laboratories involved in chromosomal studies and prenatal diagnosis. These are not listed here, partly to save space, but also because any interested clinician will find out personally the best channels of referral. In addition, the 'official' centre may not invariably be the most appropriate: thus, a paediatric neurologist especially involved with muscular dystrophies may be in a better position to give genetic advice than a geneticist without first-hand experience of the field.

In the USA the number of centres involved in genetic counselling is much greater and many do not have a clearly defined and secure service basis. A useful world-wide directory of Genetic Services has been produced by the National Foundation, White Plains, New York 10605, USA and is available from them free.

Lay Societies involved with Inherited Diseases

Few genetic disorders now seem to be without their own society, and these often produce helpful information for patients and their families (and for their doctors!) which may be extremely useful in conjunction with genetic counselling. Many families find the support given by such lay groups valuable, while raising money for research and pressing for adequate services are also valuable functions.

On the other hand, it has to be remembered that many families do *not* wish to be associated with lay groups, and it is important that clinicians involved in providing genetic counselling do not become so closely identified with such groups as to prevent them providing an equal service to the majority of families not involved with them.

The following list for the UK is undoubtedly incomplete and further information and corrections will be welcomed.

UK
Association to Combat Huntington's Chorea,
Lyndhurst, Lower Hampton Road, Sunbury-on-Thames, Surrey.

Association for Spina Bifida and Hydrocephalus,
Tavistock House North, Tavistock Square, London WC1H 9HJ

Down's Children's Association,
Quinborne Centre, Ridgacre Road, Quinton Road, Birmingham B32 QT4.

The Cystic Fibrosis Research Trust,
5 Blyth Road, Bromley, Kent BR1 3RS.

The Coeliac Society of the United Kingdom,
PO Box 181, London NW2 2QY.

Brittle Bone Society,
63 Byron Crescent, Dundee BB3 6SS.

The Haemophilia Society,
PO Box 9, 16 Trinity Street, London SE1 1DE.

The Friedreich's Ataxia Group,
Bolsover House, 8/16 Clipstone Street, London W1.

Muscular Dystrophy Group of Great Britain,
Nattrass House, 35 Macaulay Road, Clapham, London SW4 0QP.

Association for Research into Restricted Growth,
24 Pinchfield, Maple Cross, Rickmansworth, Hertfordshire.

The British Retinitis Pigmentosa Society,
24 Palmer Close, Redhill, Surrey RH1 4BX.

UK Thalassaemia Society,
107 Nightingale Lane, London N.8.

USA
A published list of the numerous North American lay societies involved
with genetic disease, as well as other useful information, can be obtained
from:

The National Clearinghouse for Human Genetic Diseases (Dept of Health,
Education and Welfare), 1776 East Jefferson Street, Rockville, Maryland
20852, USA.

Prenatal Diagnosis of Metabolic Diseases (p. 90)
Information can be obtained for the UK from: Prenatal Diagnosis Group,
Regional Cytogenetics Centre, Southmead Hospital, Westbury-on-Trym,
Bristol BS10 5NB, and for the USA from the National Clearinghouse for
Human Genetic Diseases (*see above*).

Index

Bold type indicates a major heading among multiple entries.